Otological Significance of the Round Window

Advances in Oto-Rhino-Laryngology

Vol. 33

Series Editor
C. R. Pfaltz, Basel

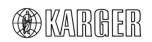

⊕ KARGER

S. Karger · Basel · München · Paris · London · New York · Tokyo · Sydney

Otological Significance of the Round Window

Yasuya Nomura

Professor and Chairman, Department of Otolaryngology, University of Tokyo

78 figures (10 in colour) and 12 tables, 1984

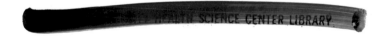

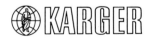

KARGER

S. Karger · Basel · München · Paris · London · New York · Tokyo · Sydney

Advances in Oto-Rhino-Laryngology

National Library of Medicine, Cataloging in Publication
     Nomura, Yasuya, 1932 –
     Otological significance of the round window/
     Yasuya Nomura. — Basel; New York: Karger, 1984.
     (Advances in oto-rhino-laryngology; v. 33)
     Includes index.
     1. Cochlea   I. Title   II. Series
     W1 AD701 v. 33 [WV 250 N8110]
     ISBN 3–8055–3806–5

Drug Dosage
     The authors and the publisher have exerted every effort to ensure that drug selection and dosage set forth in this text are in accord with current recommendations and practice at the time of publication. However, in view of ongoing research, changes in government regulations, and the constant flow of information relating to drug therapy and drug reactions, the reader is urged to check the package insert for each drug for any change in indications and dosage and for added warnings and precautions. This is particularly important when the recommended agent is a new and/or infrequently employed drug.

Contents

Preface

The oval window and the round window demarcate the middle ear from the inner ear. In this sense, these two windows are of equal importance. It is known that the oval window has a stapes, and a great deal of research has been done on the anatomy, physiology, pathology and diseases pertaining to this window. The round window, however, has been rather ignored.

Anatomically speaking, the round window is located deep inside the round window niche which opens posteriorly, inferiorly and laterally in the tympanic cavity. This seems to be the reason why the round window has remained obscure.

Recently, it has been found that diseases of the round window, especially round window ruptures, are not rare and that hearing loss and vertigo are experienced by patients with round window ruptures. It has been proved that early and appropriate treatment is effective.

It has also been discovered that drugs can permeate via the round window membrane to the labyrinth. Heretofore, the damage caused by this permeation has been emphasized.

The experiments described in this volume, however, show that β-receptor blockers, antibiotics and steroids can easily pass through the round window membrane. In the future, it is expected that treatments of labyrinthine diseases will be conducted via the round window membrane.

I decided some years ago that the study of diseases of the round window and clarification of the role of this window in treating ear diseases would be an important contribution to otorhinolaryngology. It has been my great pleasure to study this subject, the opportunity for which was given in 1982 by President *Takashi Tsuiki* of the 83rd Annual Meeting of the Japanese Society of Oto-Rhino-Laryngology.

This book would not have been possible without the help of my colleagues in the Department of Otolaryngology, University of Tokyo. Acknowledgment is made especially to Associate Professor *I. Kawabata*, Assistant Professors *M. Oda*, *T. Futaki*, and *T. Fukaya*, Drs. *T. Harada*, *K. Shima*, and *T. Okuno*.

I also extend my thanks to Professor *K. Hoshino*, Department of Anatomy, University of Kyoto, and Professor *O. Tanaka*, Department of Anatomy, Shimane Medical College, for chapter 2, Professor *Y. Wada* and Dr. *Y. Ono*, Department of Physics, University of Tokyo, for pp. 41–43 chapter 5, Professor Emeritus *T. Uemura*, Drs. *Y. Ohba* and *M. Noguchi*, Department of Precision Machinery Engineering, University of Tokyo, for pp. 72–74 chapter 5, and Dr. *T. Miyata*, Director of Japan Biomedial Material Research Center, for pp. 61–63 chapter 5.

Professor *C.R. Pfaltz*, Editor of *Advances in Oto-Rhino-Laryngology*, gave me a great deal of helpful advice. I would also like to thank Ms. *S. Schmidt* for checking the English translation and Ms. *H. Miyazaki* for typing the manuscript. This study was supported by a Research Grant for Specific Diseases from the Ministry of Health and Welfare's Acute Profound Deafness Research Committee of Japan, and Grants-in-Aid for Scientific Research 57440075 and for Developmental Scientific Research 56870010 from the Ministry of Education of Japan.

I will be very happy if this booklet is of use to doctors in their daily clinical practice as well as in basic research.

Yasuya Nomura

Introduction

Since the publication of *Corti's* famous thesis on the structure of the inner ear in 1841 quite a few important monographs have appeared presenting the morphological aspects of the hearing organ. The round window however has remained one of the scientifically neglected parts of the inner ear. The monograph of *Yasuya Nomura* fills this gap and its scientific standard is far above an ordinary state of the art review on a highly specialized topic. The volume covers a wide range of subjects relating not only to the morphology but also to physiology, biochemistry, pathophysiology and clinical pathology of this little organ – ignored for so many years and yet so important both to the research worker in the laboratory and the clinician.

C.R. Pfaltz, Basel

1. Brief History of Studies of the Cochlear Window

The cochlear window is said to have been detected and designated by *Fallopius* (1523–1563), *Vidius* (1500–1567), *Ingrassias* (1510–1580) and others. However, it has been given various names, and such words as 'posterior foramen' (*Vesalius*, 1514–1564), 'tortuous round window', 'curved window' (*Casserius*, 1561–1616), 'oval window' (*Thomas Willis*, 1612–1675), and 'circular window' (*Valsalva*, 1666–1723) have been used. In this book, the author will use the term 'the round window'.

The first researcher to describe the round window in detail was *Antonio Scarpa* (1747–1832) of Modena. In 1772, he observed the round window and the round window membrane and described their structures (fig. 1a, b). *Scarpa* was said to have borne a strong resemblance to *Napoleon* (1769–1821) in his adolescence, and another publication by *Scarpa* includes his portrait (fig. 2).

It had already been pointed out by *Cassebohm* (1700–1743) that the round window took on a triangular shape, and *Scarpa*, making similar observations, mentioned that the outside appearance of the round window of a fetus differed from that of an adult, the former showing a round or oval shape.

It was *Casserius'* discovery that the round window is not open but is occluded by a membrane. *Scarpa* added to this by pointing out that the membrane is not flat but is rather conical. *Haller* stated that this window has the appearance of a canal rather than a simple foramen. *Scarpa* said that sound is conveyed to the inner ear via a space in this canal, and that the relationship between the canal and the round window membrane resembles that between the external auditory meatus and the tympanic membrane. He thought, therefore, that it would be appropriate to call the round window membrane 'tympano secundario', or the secondary tympanum.

The cochlear window is generally referred to as the round window. In Japan, the word *enso* (meaning "round window") was used in an early publication, *Kaitai Shinsho (The New Book on Anatomy)*, in 1774. *Kaitai Shinsho* is a Japanese translation of *Ontleedkundige Tagelen* (a Dutch publication)

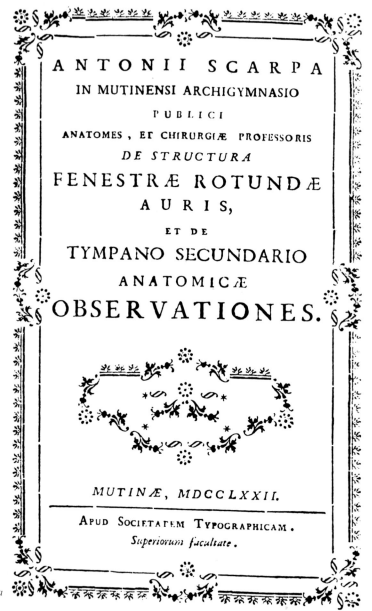

ANTONII SCARPA

IN MUTINENSI ARCHIGYMNASIO

PUBLICI

ANATOMES, ET CHIRURGIÆ PROFESSORIS

DE STRUCTURA

FENESTRÆ ROTUNDÆ

AURIS,

ET DE

TYMPANO SECUNDARIO

ANATOMICÆ

OBSERVATIONES.

MUTINÆ, MDCCLXXII.

APUD SOCIETATEM TYPOGRAPHICAM.

Superiorum facultate.

1a

Fig. 1.a The original work of *Scarpa*, published in 1772, 141 pages, 21 × 14 cm (Collection of the Research Institute of Labor and Sciences). *b* Illustrations seen in *Scarpa's* book. This is one of two such illustrations in the work (Tab. 1). An enlargement of Fig. IX is seen on the bottom left-hand side.

Tab. I

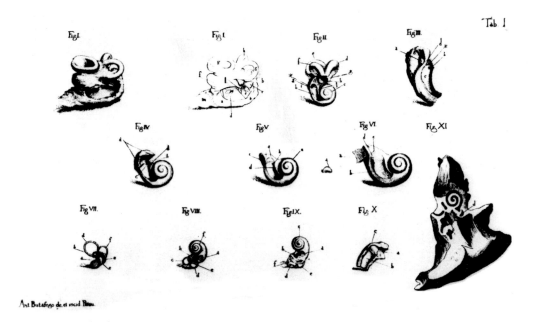

Ant. Butafogo de. et incid. Patav.

FIG. IX.

Idem atque superior figura oftendit Suis labyrinthus.

a. Feneftra rotunda potius triangulari figura.
b. Feneftra ovalis.
c. Cochleæ gyri.
d. Canalis femicircularis major.
e. Minimus.
f. Minor.

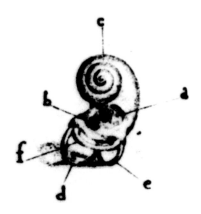

1b

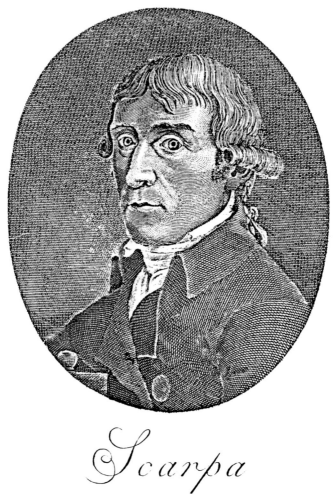

$\mathcal{Scarpa}$

Fig. 2. Portrait of *Scarpa*. Saggio di Osservazioni e d'Esperienze sulle principali Malattie degli Occhi (1802 edition) translated as 'Observations and Experiences on the Principle Maladies of the Eyes' (Collection of Kodansha Classic Medical Library).

containing anatomical charts with Dutch explanations. This book was translated by *Ryotaku Maeno* and *Genpaku Sugita* in 1771–1774. The physiology and anatomy terminology section in the first edition of a German-Japanese medical dictionary, published in 1881 by the Jiyu-jizai Dokuritsu Fuki Do, shows the same word, 'enso', which was probably taken directly from *Kaitai Shinsho*.

Sei enso (literally, 'true round window') first appeared in 1893 in an anatomical publication, *Kaibo Ranyo Ku (The Nine Key Points of Anatomy)* by *Kazuyoshi Taguchi*, who described the *sei enso* leading to the *kagyu kaku* (cochlea) and occluded by a membrane named *fuku komaku* (the secondary tympanum).

Basel Nomina Anatomica (BNA, 1895) employed the word 'fenestra cochlea' as opposed to the so-called round window; thus the Japanese name became *kagyu so* (cochlear window). Since then, both Jena Nomina Anatomica (JNA, 1935) and Nomina Anatomica Parisiensia (PNA, 1955) show no changes in the use of the word; in Japan, too, the term *kagyu so* has been used continuously in anatomical terminology up to the present time.

In 1556, *Coiter* (1534–1600?), and in 1683, *Du Verney* (1648–1730) pointed out that sound is transmitted to the inner ear both via the oval window and the round window. *Schelhammer* [1684] defined sound as being transmitted to the inner ear only via the round window. Later, however, the concept of the function of the round window as the 'escape route' for the pressure necessary to induce vibrations of the fluid enclosed in the inner ear gradually became accepted.

As a natural consequence, the question arose of whether changes in hearing occur when the round window becomes obstructed. There have been numerous reports from the clinical point of view. *Habermann* [1901] stated, for example, that in cases where the round window was occluded by ossification, the hearing showed no sign of deterioration. However, the degree of occlusion was not verified. *Oppikofer* [1917] reported on 2 cases in which the round windows were obstructed by adipose tissue, and stated that the hearing in the 2 cases was normal.

Communication between the cochlea and the cranial cavity involves the cochlear aqueduct, the perineural space and the perivascular space; *Ranke* et al. [1952] used the general term 'the third window' for all these organs. According to *Groen and Hoogland* [1958], in cases where the round window becomes obstructed due to otosclerosis, hearing via bone conduction deteriorates hardly at all in the low frequency region, provided that the cochlear aqueduct and the inferior cochlear vein remain open. The same report, however, states that the higher the frequency, the less the leak from the scala tympani to these organs. This increases the impedance, and, as a result, a deterioration of bone conduction at 6 dB per 1 octave will be seen. From the phylogenetic viewpoint, the above-mentioned report stirs one's curiosity in light of the fact that prior to the appearance of the round window, the communication between the cochlea and the cranial cavity was conducted largely via the foramen perilymphaticum.

Several experiments have been conducted in which some effect on hearing was detected in cases where the round window was obstructed. However, *Gisselsson and Richter's* [1955] review of documents from the past shows that there is a lack of consistency in these experiments. Of 25 documents on changes in hearing, the hearing was reported to be lowered in 12, to be improved in 9 and to show no change in 4. One of the reasons for such diverse results could be differences in the type of obstruction.

Tonndorf and Tabor [1962] completely obstructed the round window of a cat with silicon and cement. Their report on this experiment shows that when the cochlear aqueduct was open, there was no significant change observed in either air conduction or bone conduction. *Weber-Liel* [1876], *Kobrak* [1949] and others carried out experiments using the round window membrane in humans. *Kobrak* studied various physiological characteristics of the membrane using isolated round window specimens taken from the temporal bone.

Békésy [1936] stated that if the tympanic membrane and the auditory ossicles are lost, sound will be heard differently. Specifically, he said that since the sound pressure from the oval window to the round window in such a case is greater than normal, sound would be heard in inverted phase. Several methods of compensating for loss of tympanic membrane and auditory ossicles have been reported. The method of transmitting vibrations from the tympanic membrane to the round window by means of tympanoplasty has been reported by *Stevenson* [1961], *García-Ibáñez* [1959] and others. The method of forming the upper portion of the tympanic cavity by opening up the vicinity of the round window to the external auditory meatus has been advocated by *Sato* [1963] for those cases in which ear discharge persists due to lesions such as sinus tympani or hypotympanic cells.

The round window used to become a clinical issue mainly in conjunction with labyrinthitis, when it extended into the inner ear. Through the discovery and popularization of antibiotics, however, such cases of labyrinthitis have been diminishing drastically. On the other hand, microscopes have been introduced to surgery in the otological field, and surgical procedures have been used to eliminate obstruction of the round window caused by anomaly, otosclerosis and so on. Nevertheless, this trend has not attracted widespread attention.

Recently, it has been shown that the round window membrane can be ruptured. Furthermore, the frequency of such damage is quite high. The

symptoms and signs are at times similar to those of sudden deafness, and progressive or fluctuating hearing loss may also be reported. Dizziness and disequilibrium occur in many cases. In the examination and diagnosis of clinical
cases suffering from such symptoms, it would be well to bear in mind the possibility of rupture of the round window membrane and/or of the oval window. The round window membrane has thus begun to attract the attention
of clinicians more than ever before.

2. Phylogenesis

The inner ear is largely occupied by the inner ear fluids, i.e., the endolymph and perilymph. This is true of the cochlea and also of the vestibulum and semicircular canals. However, from a phylogenetical viewpoint, the vestibulum and semicircular canals appear first, followed by the formation of the perilymphatic duct, which is concurrent with the time when the inner ear begins to play a role as an auditory organ. The perilymphatic system has a much more important function in the cochlea than in the vestibulum and semicircular canals.

As indicated in figure 3, the primitive inner ear is made up of the semicircular canals, the utricle and the saccule, and is surrounded by the perilymphatic system which contains the connective tissue. The primitive inner ear has no organ of hearing. At the next stage, as differentiation progresses, a new sense organ, the lagena, is formed on a bulge rising from the saccule. The perilymphatic system attached to this new sense organ is devoid of connective tissue (fig. 4). This newly developed space is called the perilymphatic duct. The perilymphatic duct has two windows: one contains the columella or stapes, and the other is occluded by a membrane which lies at the far end. This latter window is the round window. When sound waves are transported to the columella or stapes, massive movements of the perilymph take place, vibrations of which are received by the newly developed sense organ.

Fishes are classified into two groups according to the function of sound transmission. One group is the *Ostariophysi* which have an organ called the sinus impar which corresponds to the perilymphatic duct. The air bladder contracts and expands, responding to vibrations produced by water. These movements are transmitted to the tripus (triangular bone) which is adjacent to the air bladder and then to the sinus impar. Finally, the vibrations are received by the saccule and the lagena. The other group, the Non-ostariophysi, lack such an organ [*Tumarkin, 1948*].

A specific sound transmission system is formed in the tadpole stage of the frog *(Rana)*. This system transmits oscillations of the air within the lungs. A membrane resembling the tympanic membrane is formed in the bronchi

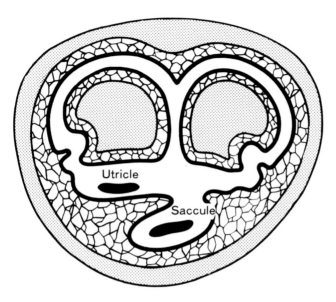

Fig. 3. The primitive inner ear. The perilymphatic system surrounds the labyrinth, but the perilymphatic duct is not yet seen [*de Burlet*, 1928/1929].

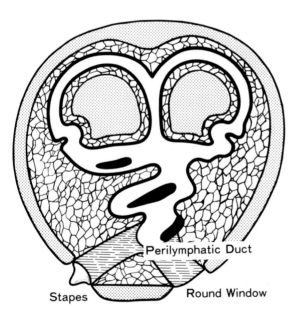

Fig. 4. The developed inner ear. The perilymphatic duct is formed, and the stapes and the round window membrane can be seen on either side [*de Burlet*, 1928/1929].

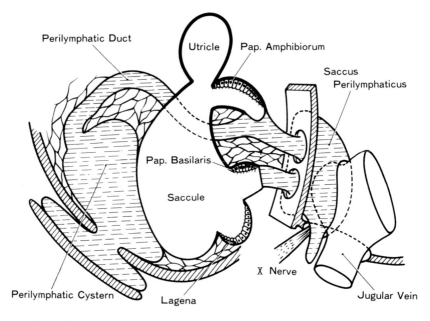

Fig. 5. The perilymphatic system of the frog *(Rana)*. Besides the lagena, there are two sensory epithelia, the papilla amphibiorum and the papilla basilaris. Two perilymphatic ducts join at the cranial cavity, and the perilymphatic sac touches the jugular vein. The round window is lacking [*de Burlet,* 1928/1929].

area, and short rods originating from the membrane form the infantile columella, which reaches the round window. The columella penetrates the root of the aorta at both its ends and is covered by the aortic endothelium. During the time which a tadpole metamorphoses into a frog, the columella of the middle ear in the adult form becomes associated with the oval window, and the temporary apparatus of hearing which was formed in the bronchi area disappears [*Portmann,* 1976].

The frog has two perilymphatic ducts which join at the cranial cavity to form the perilymphatic sac, a part of which passes, together with the jugular vein and the vagus nerve, through the jugular foramen. Moreover, the perilymphatic sac lies largely adjacent to the jugular notch (fig. 5). Generally, in highly evolved land animals, the labyrinth and the cranial cavity communicate through two foramens: the endolymphatic foramen and the perilymphatic foramen. The endolymphatic sac and the perilymphatic sac grow into the cranial cavity through these foramens (fig. 6, 7).

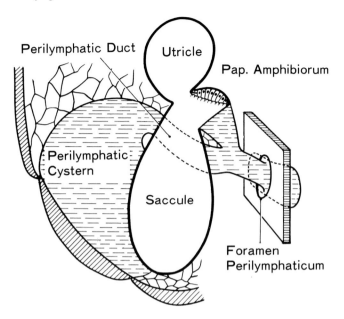

Fig. 6. The perilymphatic system of the proteus *(Olm)* [*de Burlet*, 1928/1929].

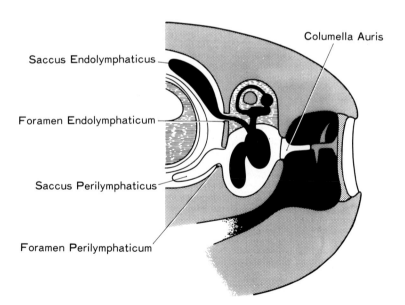

Fig. 7. The inner ear of *Reptilia*. The round window is lacking in certain reptiles [*Portmann*, 1976].

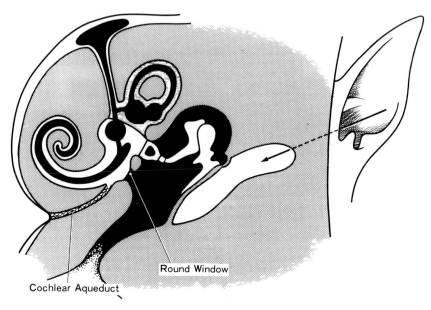

Fig. 8. The inner ear of *Mammalia* [*Portmann*, 1976].

Reptiles *(Reptilia)* are classified into two groups according to the mechanism of sound transmission. In one group, the round window membrane plays a role in adjusting changes in perilymphatic pressure as in birds *(Aves)* and mammals *(Mammalia).* The *Crocodilia* belong to this group. The *Hemidactylus* also have the round window. Land animals of the other group, such as turtles, snakes, *Amphisbaenidians* and *Sphenodon,* lack the round window membrane [*Turner,* 1980] (fig. 7).

In a number of reptiles, birds and mammals, the area where the cranial cavity and the inner ear communicate is narrow, the perilymphatic foramen is atrophied into the cochlear aqueduct and the endolymphatic duct is thin. In spite of the stenosis of the perilymphatic foramen, a new window opens into the tympanic cavity: this newly formed window is the round window by which changes in perilymphatic pressure remain controlled [*Portmann,* 1976] (fig. 8).

Figure 9 shows the structure of the inner ear of the *Trionyx sinensis.* The inner ear of reptiles is made up of the utricle, semicircular canals, saccule, lagena and papilla basilaris. A part of the perilymphatic cavity protrudes through the perilymphatic foramen surrounded by bones and cartilage into the cranial cavity to form the perilymphatic sac.

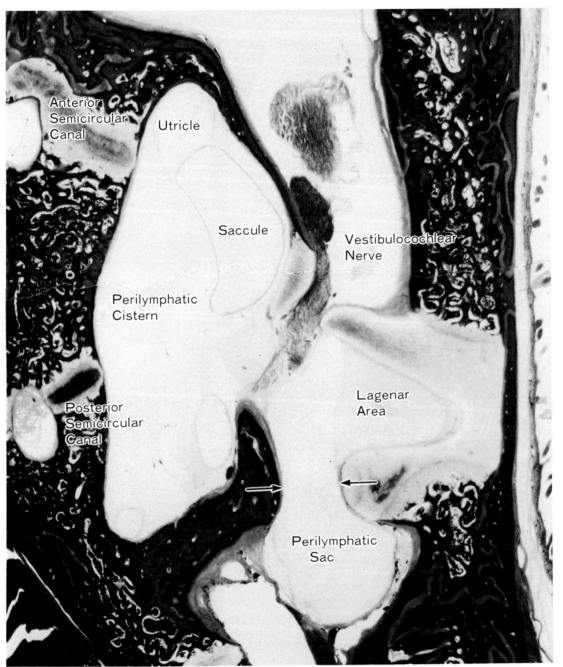

Anterior Semicircular Canal

Utricle

Saccule

Vestibulocochlear Nerve

Perilymphatic Cistern

Posterior Semicircular Canal

Lagenar Area

Perilymphatic Sac

Fig. 9. The inner ear of *Trionyx sinensis.* The perilymphatic sac protrudes through the perilymphatic foramen (area between two arrows) into the cranial cavity.

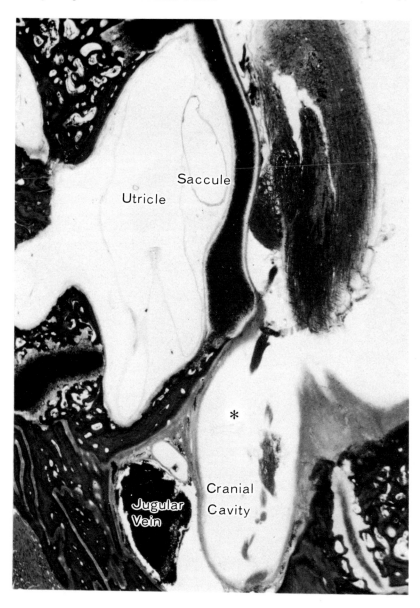

Fig. 10. The inner ear of *Trionyx sinensis.* The perilymphatic sac (*) is seen in the cranial cavity.

The perilymphatic sac, which is also called the periotic sac, is attached to the jugular vein (fig. 9, 10). Figure 9 shows the nerve coming from the cranial cavity into the inner ear. However, the sensory epithelium is not observed and only a small number of nerve fibers are seen in the lagenar area. Figure 10 shows the cranial cavity attached to the perilymphatic sac which projects into the cranial cavity.

3. Embryology

The following is a review of the embryology of the inner ear in a human fetus based on the literature. The growth of the auditory placode is detected in the 2-mm crown-rump length (CRL) stage and the otic vesicle in the 3-mm CRL stage. In the CRL 6.3–6.7 mm stage, the endolymphatic sac is beginning to form, and in the 8–9 mm stage, the original semicircular canals are seen. In the 12-mm stage, the endolymphatic duct and the endolymphatic sac are discernible. In the 30-mm stage, the cochlea has one and a half turns.

As for the endolymphatic cavity and the perilymphatic cavity, the former grows first, and the latter does not appear until considerably later. In a fetus of CRL 9 mm, the original epithelium is wrapped in mesenchymal tissue, which changes into precartilage at 16 mm [*Streeter*, 1918] and later becomes the hyaline cartilage. In a fetus of 30–40 mm, the perilymphatic cavity appears for the first time, and this is what is called 'perilymphatic cistern' [*Foley*, 1931]. In the 43-mm stage, the growth of the scala tympani is observed [*Streeter*, 1918]. As the fetus develops to CRL 50 mm, the scala vestibuli can be observed: at the same time, the cochlea develops to two and a half turns. In the 70–80 mm stage, the perilymphatic cavity of the semicircular canals arises, and in the 130-mm stage, the complete forms of the scala vestibuli and the scala tympani appear and the development of the helicotrema begins.

The rudimentary stapes is observed in the 7-mm fetus [*Cauldwell and Anson*, 1942]. When the fetus is CRL 22–23 mm, it becomes precartilage, and the timing coincides with the beginning of the development of the round window. In the 27-mm stage, the syncytium cells begin to condense [*Waltner*, 1945]. In the 45-mm stage, this condensation gradually progresses and begins to take on the shape of the round window membrane, though it is still impossible to distinguish it from the loose syncytium of the round window niche. At the 110-mm stage, a layer of enchondral cells begins to cover the inner aspect of the intermediate layer of the round window membrane. As in phylogenesis, the endolymphatic cavity appears first, followed by the

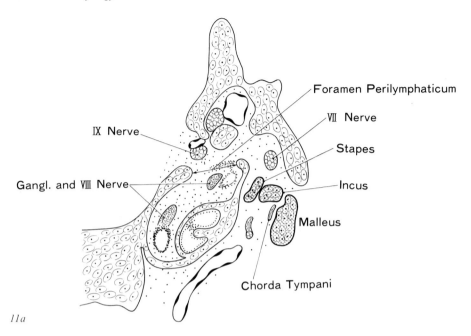

Foramen Perilymphaticum

VII Nerve

Stapes

IX Nerve

Incus

Gangl. and VIII Nerve

Malleus

Chorda Tympani

11a

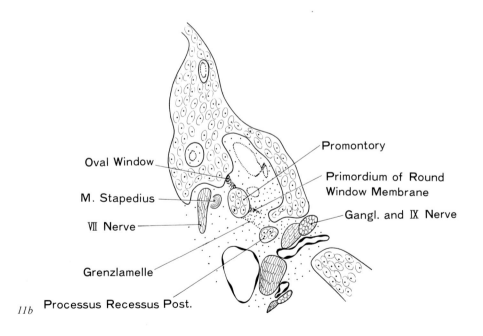

Promontory

Oval Window

Primordium of Round
Window Membrane

M. Stapedius

Gangl. and IX Nerve

VII Nerve

Grenzlamelle

11b Processus Recessus Post.

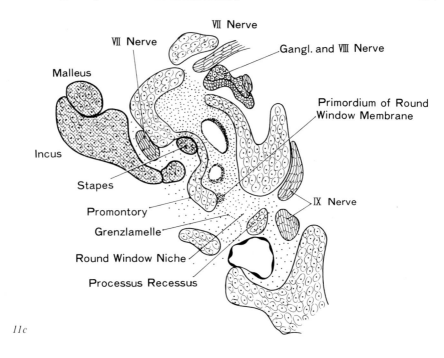

11c

perilymphatic cavity: the round window membrane also begins to be formed at about this period.

To describe the development of the round window niche, I would like to refer to figure 11, taken from *Frick* [1953]. As this figure shows, the round window niche is the communication route connecting the middle ear and the cranial cavity.

A study was made by the author of the genesis of the round window membrane in 9 human fetuses. The CRL (mm) and the ages in weeks (in parentheses) of the 9 fetuses are as follows: 20.7 mm (8 weeks), 50.5 (9), 60.0 (10), 72.0 (11), 84.0 (12), 155.0 (17), 184.0 (20), 205.0 (22) and 313.0 (36). These fetuses were fixed in formalin and embedded in paraffin, and a series of sections 5 µm in thickness were prepared (HE staining).

CRL 20.7-mm Stage (8-Week-Old Fetus). This stage is equivalent to the 22nd phase in the Carnegie system of classification. The otic capsule is precartilaginous and its contour is vague. However, it is divided into the pars cochlearis and the pars canalicularis, and mesenchymal tissue occupying the space between their divisions connects the tympanic portion and the menin-

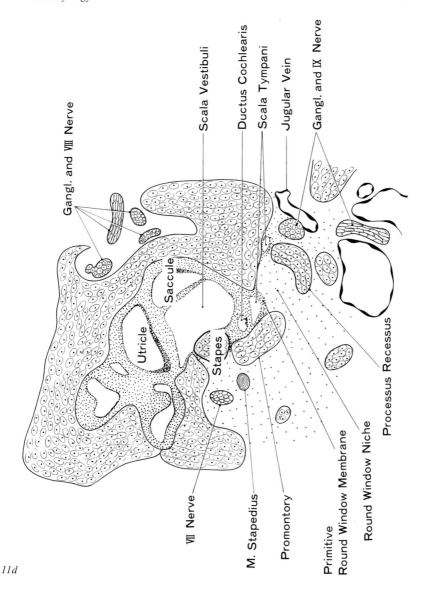

11d

Fig. 11. The development of the round window niche of man [*Frick*, 1953]. *a* Fetus, CRL 27-mm stage. *b* Fetus, CRL 37-mm stage. *c* Fetus, CRL 42-mm stage. *d* Fetus, CRL 68-mm stage.

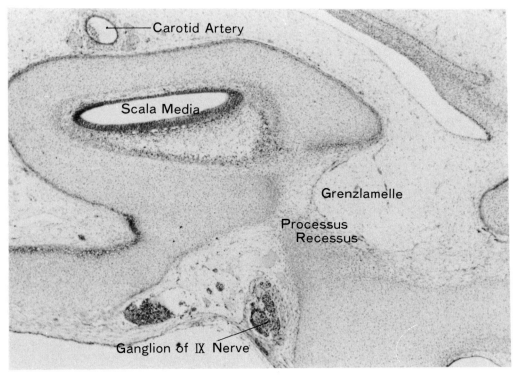

12a

geal portion. This space is called hiatus tympanomeningealis [*Bast and Anson*, 1952], or recessus scalae tympani [*Frick*, 1953]. The cochlear canal has already formed a cavity inside the cochlea at this stage, but the perilymphatic cavity is not yet completed. The vicinity of its foramen, the perilymphatic foramen, has an area that has been partially reticulated. The outside forms the boundary from the promontory through the hiatus to the external aspect of the semicircular canals, consisting of cells which are well stained by the basic component of HE stain. This dense cell group differs clearly from the gelatinous tissue inside the tympanic cavity, and the nuclei are thin and long. This group is called 'Grenzlamelle' [*Frick*, 1953] and is thought to contribute to the formation of the future round window membrane.

CRL 50.5-mm Stage (9-Week-Old Fetus). The internal wall of the perilymphatic foramen, as compared to the external wall, is markedly hypertrophic posteriorly, and the internal portion partly expands downward to

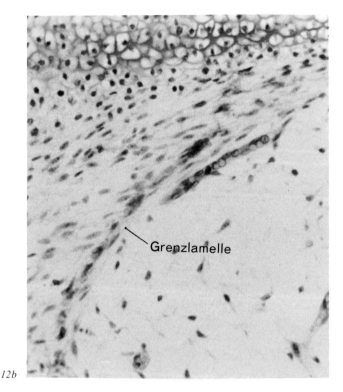

12b

Fig. 12. a The formation of the cochlear duct is seen, but the perilymphatic cavity has not yet been formed. Grenzlamelle is observed outside of the processus recessus and near the perilymphatic foramen. *b* Grenzlamelle: enlarged view of figure 12a. Grenzlamelle is made up of a group of cells with a thin and long nucleus. It lies adjacent to the otic capsule cartilage, though it is clearly different from the gelatinous tissue occupying the tympanic cavity.

become the processus recessus anterior. There is also a cartilage growing from the vicinity of the prominentia utriculo-ampullaris inferior of the semicircular canals to the bottom edge of the perilymphatic foramen anterosuperiorly, surrounding the inside from the bottom. This is the processus recessus posterior; all these will be fused in the future to form the crista semilunaris. The scala tympani shows loose reticular tissues and the clear existence of the intrachondrial membrane; the cavity, however, has not been formed yet. The mesenchymal tissue medial to the Grenzlamelle fades away from the promontory toward the processus recessus posterior, and at the same time the gelatinous tissue inside the tympanic cavity approaches the perilymphatic foramen (fig. 12).

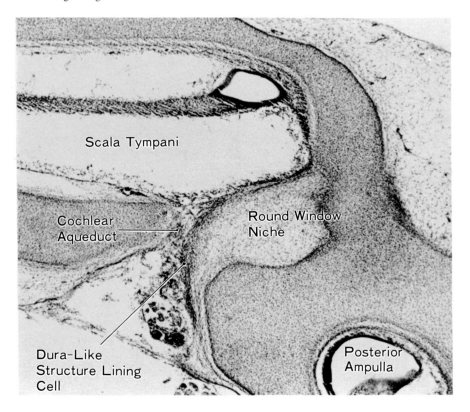

Fig. 13. CRL 72.0-mm stage. Dura-like structure lining cell joins the original round window membrane along the cochlear aqueduct.

CRL 60.0-mm Stage (10-Week-Old Fetus). The ground substance of the cartilage of the inner ear stains easily, and the structure showing characteristics of the perichondrium is clearly seen on the surface. The canal is beginning to form in the scala tympani, and, concurrently, a decrease in the reticular tissue is observed. The mesothelium of the perilymphatic cavity extends inside the round window membrane. The mesenchymal tissue of the Grenzlamelle has become looser, and the intracellular spaces are wider. The cell has a long cytoplasm, existing parallel to the round window membrane, and some of the cells become the intermediate layer of the round window membrane. The processus recessus anterior and the processus recessus posterior have not yet been united.

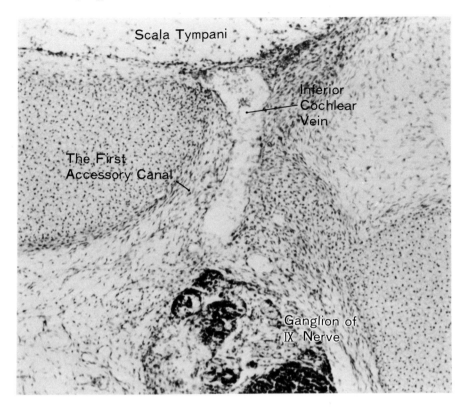

Fig. 14. CRL 72.0-mm stage. Inferior cochlear vein and the first accessory canal.

CRL 72.0-mm Stage (11-Week-Old Fetus). The contour of the perichondrium has become even clearer. On the other hand, the contour of the Grenzlamelle is vague, and the mesenchymal tissue is becoming loose, showing larger intercellular spaces. The original cochlear aqueduct moves from the endocranial cavity to the inner side of the round window. The cochlear aqueduct has a bundle of spindle cells moving toward the round window membrane. This is what *Waltner* [1945] called the dura-like structure lining cell, and it is linked to the dura mater (fig. 13, 14). Furthermore, there is the syncytium outside this dura-like structure lining cell, which is destined to be cartilagified and to serve as the support of the cochlear aqueduct.

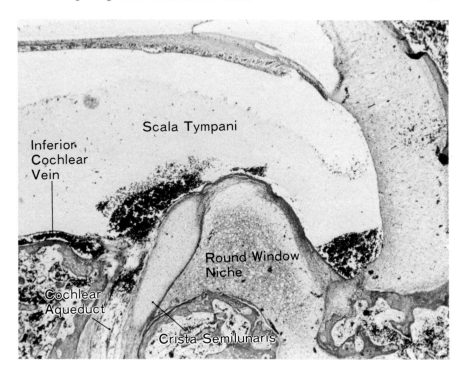

Fig. 15. CRL 155.0-mm stage. The cochlear aqueduct is seen along the crista semilunaris.

CRL 84.0-mm Stage (12-Week-Old Fetus). The mesenchymal tissues which were medial to and adjacent to the Grenzlamelle have all but disappeared, and the gelatinous tissues inside the tympanic cavity occupy their space. The round window membrane is partially covered by the syncytium originating from the niche and is believed to contribute to the formation of the membrane.

CRL 155.0-mm Stage (17-Week-Old Fetus). The cartilaginous wall of the round window niche has been ossified except for the bottom part, i.e., the cartilaginous processus recessus which separates the round window membrane from the cochlear aqueduct (fig. 15). The bony wall of the labyrinth is made up of three layers. The inner (endosteal) layer is thin, and the middle layer attains remarkable development at this stage, showing the growth of intrachondral bone. The outer (periosteal) layer does not develop at this stage. The round window membrane is convex to the scala tympani, near the

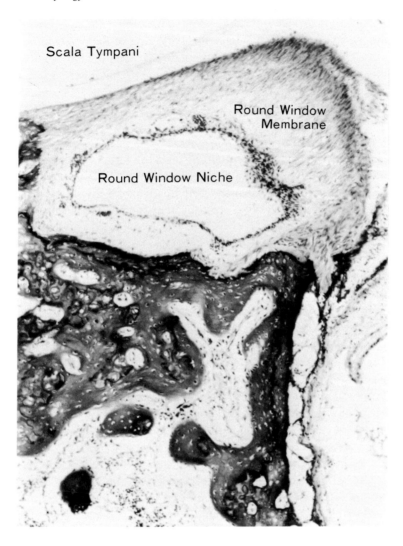

Fig. 16. CRL 205.0-mm stage. Pneumatization begins in the round window niche, and the round window membrane becomes thin and covered with an epithelial layer of mucous membrane.

superior margin of the round window. The round window membrane appears to be shaped concurrent with ossification of the otic capsule. The cochlear aqueduct is surrounded by the cartilage, with the dura periosteum running inside it. However, the dura periosteum does not participate in the round window membrane. The cavity of the cochlear aqueduct is filled with loose reticular tissues.

CRL 184.0-mm Stage (20-Week-Old Fetus). Ossification of the processus recessus is progressing, and it is attaining the adult form of the crista semilunaris. Ossification is observed in the large portion of the round window margin, i.e., the crista fenestrae cochleae, accompanying the division of the cochlear aqueduct and the inferior cochlear vein by the bony tissue.

CRL 205.0- and 313.0-mm Stages (22- and 36-Week-Old Fetuses). The wall of the round window niche is almost entirely ossified; the space thus enclosed is pneumatized through two-thirds of its depth and is lined by mucous membrane continuous with that of the tympanic cavity. In the same manner, the round window membrane is forming an epithelial layer of mucous membrane in its outer layer (fig. 16). Judging from the genesis of the round window in human fetuses, the round window area is associated with the communication route between the cranial cavity and the middle ear. In complete formation of this area is known as Hyrtl's fissure, and is the site of clinical problems due to the occurrence of liquorrhea. Melanocytes are seen in large quantities in the inner ear tissues, and their development is ectodermal, having a close connection with brain tissues. It is believed that a large number of melanin cells in the round window membrane and in the round window niche has also resulted from their relation with the hiatus. The collagen fibers of the round window membrane are fanned out from the crista semilunaris. This can be explained by the joining of dura-like structure lining cells, connected with the dura mater, into the round window membrane. The joined dura-like structure lining cells combine with the processus recessus and consequently adhere to the rim of the round window. Since the round window becomes enlarged as a result of the above fusion, the collagen fibers are believed to take on an arrangement extending from the crista semilunaris to the margin of the round window.

4. Round Window Niche and Round Window Membrane

It has been reported that the round window niche takes on a Gothic arch shape when viewed through the external auditory meatus [*Donaldson*, 1968]. It is apparent from observations during surgery, however, that it can actually present various shapes. Viewed directly from the removed temporal bone, its entrance is triangular in shape, as was reported by *Scarpa*. Its three sides have been designated as the anterior wall, superior wall and posterior wall (fig. 17), and the length of each of these walls in 34 ears was measured. The results are shown in table I.

In order to measure the areas of the entrance portions of the round window niches, straight-on photographs were taken by a surgical microscope, and measurements were obtained using a Luzex 500 Image Analyzer (to be described later). The average measurement for 33 ears was 2.84 mm^2. When the round window is observed from the external auditory meatus, the anterior wall appears closest, and the niche entrance portion is tallest where the anterior wall joins the superior wall. It is not possible to obtain a direct view of the niche side of the anterior wall: the niche side of the superior wall, however, can be observed partially.

The round window membrane can barely be seen: the part that can be observed, if any, is very small. It is easier to observe the round window membrane when the bony wall of the niche is removed. How much of the bony wall could be removed without destroying the round window membrane? To determine the thickness of the bony wall or the depth of the niche, the following measuring process was carried out. A perpendicular line drawn in the center of the posterior wall of the niche ran approximately through the joint of the superior and anterior walls. When we cut off the decalcified temporal bone on the plane perpendicular to the entrance to the niche including the above-described line, we found that the round window membrane too had been approximately halved by this process.

Using a section of this temporal bone, we measured the thickness of the bony wall at the point where the membrane was attached on its outer side (O) (fig. 18). To take the measurement, line O-O′ which connects the two ends

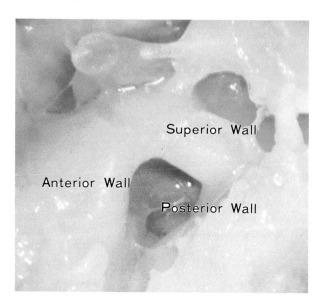

Superior Wall

Anterior Wall

Posterior Wall

Fig. 17. The round window niche (the entrance portion). A triangular shape is most frequently observed.

Table I.

	Range, mm	Average, mm
Anterior wall	0.9 – 2.1	1.5
Superior wall	0.9 – 1.7	1.3
Posterior wall	1.1 – 2.3	1.6

of the round window membrane was extended outward to point O″, and a perpendicular drawn through point P on line O″–O′ was made to touch the surface of the promontory. The value OP was thus designated to be the maximum width of the promontory. At the same time, the distance between point O and the center of the bony margin of the round window (M) was measured (OM). The measuring tool used for this purpose was a toolmaker's microscope (TM-101) with a CRT display-type data processing machine (Mitsutoyo Mfg.) attached, and the results were produced on a printer. Table II shows the results found in 10 ears.

From these figures, we can calculate how much of the margin can be dis-

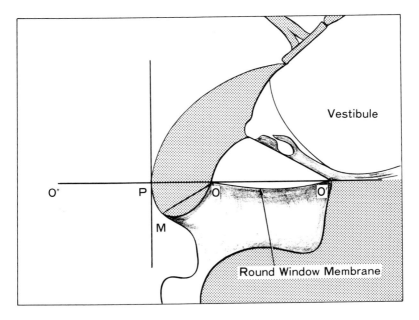

Fig. 18. Measurement of the bony margin of the round window.

Table II.

Maximum width of the promontory (OP)	1.09 – 1.63 mm (average: 1.31 mm)
Bony margin of the round window – round window membrane (OM)	0.60 – 1.58 mm (average: 0.95 mm)

sected before reaching the attachment to the membrane, at the highest part of the niche (apex of the arch) in the view from the external auditory meatus. When the anterior wall was observed from the niche side, the distance from its margin to the membrane was shortest near the point of contact between the superior wall and the anterior wall, and it became larger distally. It was concluded therefore that an area larger than the measurement taken above could be removed when the inferior portion of the anterior wall is dissected.

A study of the shape of the round window niche showed that out of 100 adult temporal bones, 67 had protruding bony margins near the entrances, which deepened the niches and thereby obstructed the views of the round window membranes. The niches of the remaining 33 ears were shallow, and it was relatively easy to observe the membranes. The measurements given in table II were obtained from only 10 decalcified temporal bones, including both relatively deep and shallow ones, which suggests that the values would have greatly varied if more temporal bones had been studied.

Membranous Structure of the Round Window Niche

It has been reported that there is mesenchymal tissue left unabsorbed in the round window niche [*Frick*, 1953; *Schicker*, 1957]. At the same time there is a theory ascribing special physiological meaning to this tissue [*Gussen*, 1978]. Membranous or reticulated structures are often viewed in the round window niche. Out of 100 ears, only 30 lacked such recognizable structures, and of the remaining 70, 13 had their niches closed off (closed type), 3 showed a reticulated structure (reticulated type) and 54 were perforated (perforated type) (fig. 19, 20). *Schicker* [1957] stated that distinguishing between the round window niche membrane and the round window membrane may be difficult when the former is of the closed type. Those with perforations can be confused with ruptured round window membranes. In fact, it is easy to mistake a perforated round window niche membrane for a ruptured round window membrane when perilymph leakage has occurred. If the round window membrane is ruptured by adding pressure experimentally to the scala tympani using a human temporal bone, a round perforation is not formed; instead, a slit running along the fibers of the intermediate layer appears.

Although further description will appear in a later chapter on rupture of the round window membrane, it should be noted here that when a membrane has a round perforation, it should be taken into consideration that it may not be the round window membrane but one consisting of connective tissue or a membrane fold. Whether this membrane can be distinguished from the round window membrane, then, is the issue. The following are the criteria for such a differentiation: (1) If a membrane has a perforation, and it is also reticulated, there is a good possibility that it is not the round window membrane. (2) The presence of melanocytes serves as a good landmark of the round window membrane. These melanocytes are scattered all over the round window membrane, especially in the area of attachment, and they can be observed under a surgical microscope (X16). It should be noted, however, that melanocytes quite often exist at the bottom of the niche adjacent to the round window membrane. (3) The round window membrane is mobile with

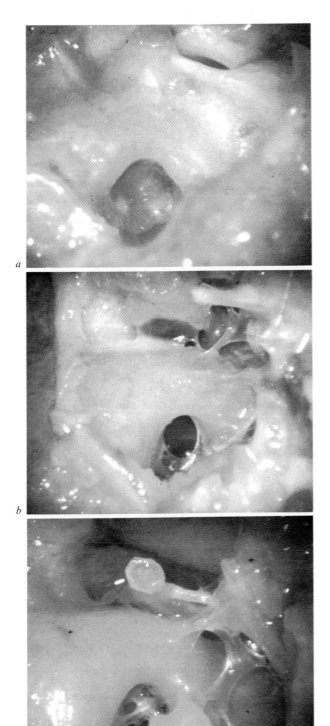

Fig. 19. Types of round window niche membrane. *a* Closed type – the niche is completely occluded. *b* Perforated type – a perforation can be seen. *c* Reticulated type – a reticulated structure can be seen.

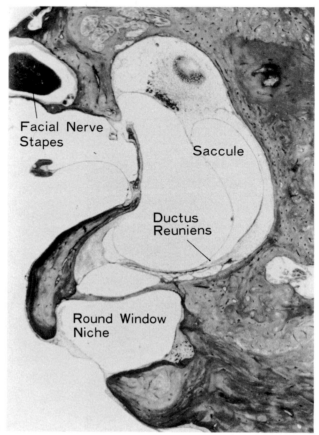

Facial Nerve

Stapes

Saccule

Ductus
Reuniens

Round Window
Niche

20a

the stapes: it bulges when the stapes is gently touched, whereas the round window niche membrane does not. (4) It is difficult to view the round window membrane from the external auditory meatus, and it is usually impossible to observe the site of rupture.

Method of Observation

How can one observe the round window niche and the round window membrane? The easiest way is to perform tympanotomy, although only part of the niche can be seen since the rest is hidden by the anterior wall. Natur-

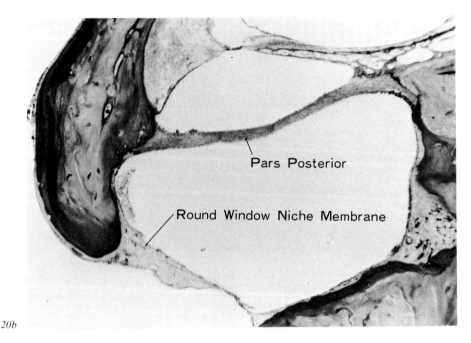

20b

Fig. 20. The round window niche membrane. *a* Vertical section of the temporal bone. *b* Enlargement of figure 20a. The scala tympani has a triangular shape.

ally, it might be possible to view part of the round window membrane, were there no membrane made up of connective tissue (fig. 21). When posterior tympanotomy is carried out, the visible portion becomes substantially larger. If the bony rim of the niche is dissected, the round window membrane becomes largely visible too (fig. 21).

Observation of the round window membrane from various angles in the temporal bone showed that observation through the space created as a result of the removal of the bony wall of the hypotympanum would be the most successful way of viewing the whole of the membrane. This method is impossible to carry out, however, in patients. Thus, observation using a needle otoscope was done as an alternative. A needle otoscope is a nonflexible, slender instrument covered by a stainless steel tube, 1.7 or 2.2 mm in outer diameter. A Selfoc rod lens, 0.7 or 1 mm in diameter, and glass fiber for illumination are stored inside. There is a prism near the tip of the needle otoscope, and this prism makes oblique or lateral viewing possible. A needle otoscope at the anterior oblique angle (60°) produces satisfactory observation of the round

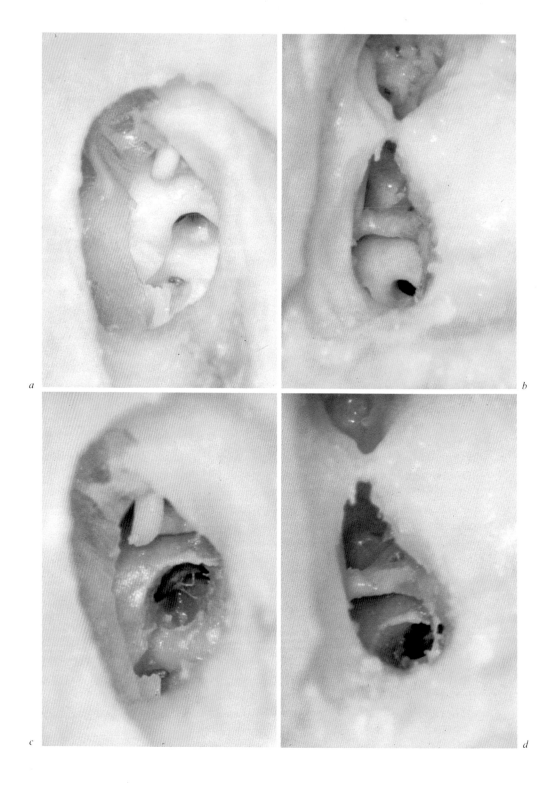

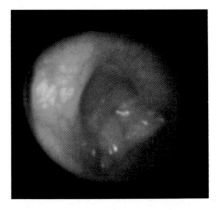

Fig. 22. The round window membrane as observed by an oblique type needle otoscope. This is a case with a large perforation as a result of chronic otitis media of the left ear. The bony annulus has not been eliminated.

window niche, and in fact this has been done in outpatients with a large perforation [*Nomura*, 1982a, b].

In order to observe the round window membrane completely, the tympanic membrane has to be elevated and the bony annulus in the posteroinferior part needs to be eliminated because insertion from the perforated area of the tympanic membrane is difficult. A needle otoscope is then inserted into the hypotympanum, with the prism side facing upwards. The round window membrane lies horizontally deep in the niche, so damage due to the insertion of the needle otoscope can be avoided (fig. 22).

Round Window Membrane

The round window membrane is located almost horizontal to the ceiling of the round window niche. In a 3- to 4-month-old fetus, the round window membrane runs parallel to the tympanic membrane and is perpendicular to the ceiling [*Tröltsch*], but it becomes horizontal just prior to birth [*Kölliker*].

Fig. 21. Observation of the round window membrane (left ear). The round window membrane has been dyed red. *a* View through the external auditory meatus. *b* View by posterior tympanotomy. *c* View through the external auditory meatus (the entrance of the niche has been eliminated). *d* View by posterior tympanotomy (the entrance of the niche has been eliminated).

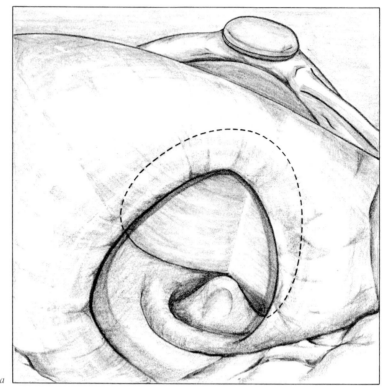

a

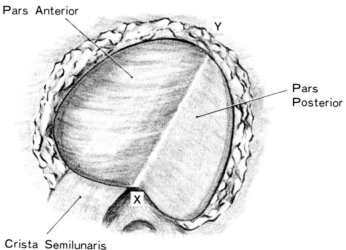

Pars Anterior

Y

Pars
Posterior

X

b   Crista Semilunaris

Fig. 23. The shape of the round window membrane. *a* It is impossible to observe the whole membrane (dotted area) unless the bony rim of the round window is dissected. *b* This membrane is divided into two sections (pars anterior and pars posterior) by line XY which runs through the center.

The round window membrane is not flat, but curves towards the scala tympani just as the tympanic membrane protrudes towards the middle ear. This is due to the structure of the part which surrounds the round window and to which the membrane is attached: i.e., bundled fibers running from the crista semilunaris to the margin of the round window. When observing the round window membrane in the temporal bone, a shallow indentation or boundary can be seen running from the crista semilunaris and almost cutting the membrane into an anterior portion, pars anterior, and a posterior portion, pars posterior (fig. 23). The pars anterior is attached to the crista semilunaris and bulges slightly towards the middle ear. Observation of vertical sections of temporal bones shows that the scala tympani is large, with a round or oval shape, and the cochlear aqueduct is open towards the inside of the crista semilunaris. The pars posterior is flat and attached to the root of the osseous spiral lamina. This makes the appearance of the scala tympani in the temporal bone specimen triangular and narrow (fig. 20b).

It should be noted that *Schaefer and Giesswein* [1926] divided the round window membrane, at a concavity to the cochlea side, into an anteroinferior portion occupying two-thirds of the membrane and a posterosuperior portion occupying the remaining one-third. In contrast, *Bast and Anson* [1952] divided the membrane into a horizontal portion in front and a vertical portion in the rear.

5. Round Window Membrane

Shape of the Round Window Membrane

The round window membrane, when removed from the temporal bone, resembles a curled hand. Its three-dimensional shape will be discussed later. Several measurements were taken of flattened round window membranes, which showed round, kidney, oval, and spatula-like shapes.

Areas, Long Diameters and Short Diameters

The areas and the long and short diameters of 50 round window membranes of adults were measured. The Luzex 500 Image Analyzer (Nippon Regulator Co., Ltd.) was used for measuring. This equipment analyzes the area, shape and number from a TV camera image, processes the data and finally outputs the results.

Round window membranes were taken out of temporal bones, compressed lightly between two slide glasses, and then examined under a light microscope. The TV images were measured and processed. 'Long diameter' indicates the maximum length obtainable by measuring the distances between two arbitrary points on the periphery of the round window membrane. 'Short diameter' refers to the maximum width obtainable of the screened image, perpendicular to the 'long diameter'. The results are shown in table III.

Round window membrane areas of 2 mm^2 [*Keith*, 1918] and 2.6 mm^2 [*Sawashima*, 1958] have been reported. As for the diameters, 2.25 × 1.0–1.25 mm [*Weber-Liel*, 1876] and 2.5 × 1.9–2.0 mm [*Beck and Bader*, 1963] have been reported. *Panse* [1897] reported maximum diameters of 2.25 mm and widths of 1–1.25 mm. It should also be noted that the areas, long diameters and short diameters of the footplates of the stapes have been measured. In order to obtain these measurements, microscopic photographs of the

Table III.

	Range	Average
Areas, mm^2	1.82 – 5.26	3.40
Long diameters, mm	1.83 – 3.25	2.30
Short diameters, mm	1.43 – 2.38	1.87

Table IV.

	Range	Average
Areas, mm^2	2.65 – 4.88	3.60
Long diameters, mm	2.67 – 3.44	3.23
Short diameters, mm	1.23 – 1.77	1.53

footplates were taken, enlarged and fed to the Luzex 500 Image Analyzer. The results of the 20 stapes measurements are shown in table IV.

The area of the oval window is slightly larger than that of the footplate of the stapes. The area and the other measurements of the oval window have been reported: 3 × 1.2 mm [*Helmholtz*, 1863], 3 × 1.5 mm [*Schwalbe, Siebenmann*], 3.7 × 2.0 mm [*Wever and Lawrence*, 1954], 3.4 mm^2 [*Sawashima*, 1958], 2.5–3.0 × 2.0 mm [*Beck and Bader*, 1963], 3.5–4.0 × 1.5–2.0 mm [*Anson*, 1961] and others.

In general, a mammal's round window membrane is larger than its oval window. The ratio of the area of the oval window to the area of the round window membrane in humans, however, is 1.3 [*Sawashima*, 1958]. The measurements taken this time gave a footplate of the stapes/round window membrane ratio of 1.06. It should be noted that this ratio is an average calculated from 20 different temporal bones.

Thickness

Using a celloidin specimen of the temporal bone, the thickness of the thinnest part of the round window membrane was measured. It was found using this method of measurement that the thinnest part (56 μm) was in the vicinity of the center of the round window membrane.

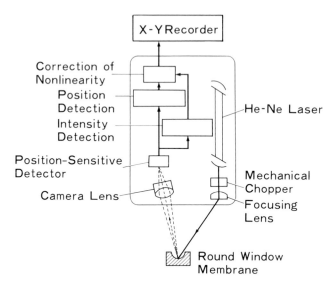

Fig. 24. Recording of the round window membrane measurements using the optical displacement meter.

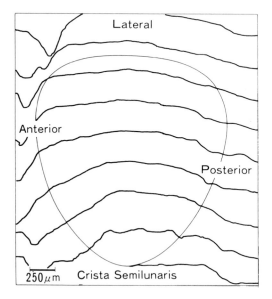

Fig. 25. The shape of the round window membrane. There is a noticeable concavity near the crista semilunaris.

Shape

Although there is a slight bulge in the tympanic cavity side, the round window membrane as a whole curves from the tympanic cavity side to the cochlea side. Two methods were employed in order to show this shape.

Method Using the Optical Displacement Meter

The optical displacement meter (Anritsu Electric Co., Ltd.) is a device which measures the size and shape of an object without directly touching it (fig. 24). A He-Ne laser beam is sharply focused through an illuminating lens and is then projected onto the surface of the object. Rays which are reflected off the surface and dispersed go through an image-forming lens and are projected onto the receptor of a light detection element. This light detection element transmits the positioning of the bundles of rays at its incidence to the receptor in the form of electric output to a computer circuit.

In measuring the round window membrane, the peripheral bone of the membrane was removed. The membrane was then placed on a stage so that its surface was nearly flat. The stage was further adjusted so that the beam would cross the longitudinal axis of the membrane. The scanning was conducted at 0.25-mm intervals on the longitudinal axis. As seen in figure 25, the resulting figure indicates that the deep niche detected near the crista semilunaris gradually becomes shallower.

Method of Reconstructing the Tissue Sections

In this method, the round window membrane was removed from the temporal bone which had been fixed in formalin. After having been embedded in paraffin, a series of sections were prepared and enlarged and measurements were taken. There was a possibility of the membrane changing its shape during this process. Reconstruction was carried out on the assumption that the whole margin of the membrane lay on the same plane.

The X axis was the line separating the membrane in halves which passed through the attachment point of the round window membrane to the crista semilunaris. The Y axis was the line perpendicular to the X axis, parallel to which were the serial sections (fig. 26). Each section was 4 μm thick. 20 sections, taken at intervals of 10 sections originally cut, were put through the HE staining method to be used as samples. These samples were enlarged and traced on graph paper to be affixed to cardboard. The affixed tracings were put together to reconstruct a model. With these samples, the sections of the membrane more or less formed parabolas. The round window membrane

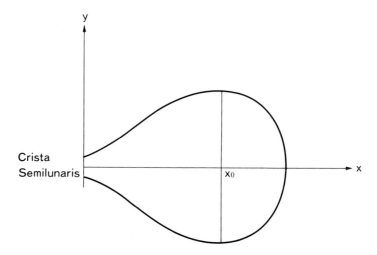

Fig. 26. The shape of the margin of the round window membrane. In this sample, the periphery can be expressed in a trigonometrical function. At X_0, this curve shows the maximum width.

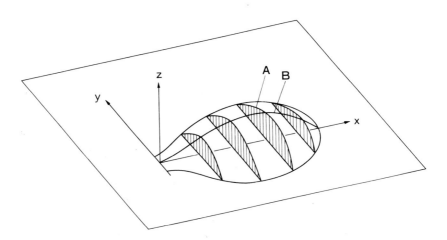

Fig. 27. The shape of the round window membrane as reconstructed by sections. Curve A is a parabola. Curve B can be expressed in two Gaussian functions.

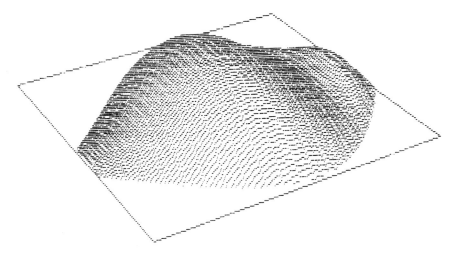

Fig. 28. Display of the round window membrane according to the approximate formula.

was approximately symmetrical on either side of the X axis. The curve can be expressed approximately in a trigonometrical function as follows:

$$f(x) = A \cos [K(x) (x - x_0)]$$
$$K(x) = K_0 \left[1 - \varepsilon^2 \left(x - x_0 - \frac{\pi}{2 K_0}\right)^2\right] \tag{1}$$

The line connecting the apexes of parabolas drawn by all sections, or the membrane, can be cut by a plane including the X axis (fig. 27). This section of the round window membrane (X axis) can be expressed approximately in two Gaussian functions as follows:

$$g(x) = \alpha e^{-(x-\beta)^2/\gamma^2} + \alpha_1 e^{-(x-\beta_1)^2/\gamma_1^2} \tag{2}$$

Thus, the expression of this round window membrane becomes

$$Z = g(x) [(f(x))^2 - y^2] \tag{3}$$

Parameters for the above formulas, incidentally, are as follows:

$A = 9.562,$ $K_0 = 0.160,$ $\varepsilon = 0.0237$
$\alpha = 0.1$ $\beta = 2.0$ $\gamma = 12.0$
$\alpha = 0.1$ $\beta_1 = 19.0$ $\gamma_1 = 1.5$

Figure 28 displays this formula.

Structure of the Round Window Membrane

Light Microscopic Findings

The round window membrane consists of three layers: the outer layer, which is continuous with the epithelial cells of the mucoperiosteum of the middle ear: the middle layer (intermediate layer), and the inner layer, which is a continuation of the cells lining the scala tympani [*Bast and Anson*, 1952] (fig. 29). The central portion of the membrane is thin, with an average thickness of 0.065 mm [*Dean and Wolff*, 1934]. Measurement for the present study recorded the thickness of this portion as 0.056 mm, becoming gradually thicker towards the periphery attached to the marginal bone of the round window membrane. Only the middle layer becomes thicker, however, with no relation to either the outer or the inner layer. The middle layer is considered to originate from either the mucoperiosteum [*Bast and Anson*, 1952] or simply the periosteum [*Dean and Wolff*, 1934] of the middle ear, bearing no connection with the inner ear tissue in either case. Embryologically speaking, the rudiment of dura mater seems to be involved in the formation of the middle layer. In the middle layer, a number of elastic fibers as well as collagen fibers are found. The elastic fibers, however, have not been observed at the circumference of the membrane, in particular near the bony margin, where the membrane becomes thick [*Harty*, 1963].

The blood vessels in the round window membrane are often seen directly beneath the outer layer. Although the direction in which blood vessels run, as well as their numbers, seems to vary from one type of animal to another [*Hata*, 1968], all of the blood vessels in this area seem to have originated from the vascular plexuses of the tympanic mucous membrane. Guinea pigs, however, sometimes show capillaries under the inner layer (fig. 44b).

The nerves in the round window membrane have already been studied in detail by *Andrzejewski* [1954] using numerous materials from both humans and dogs. These nerves predominantly run directly under the outer layer of the membrane. Plasma cells, other histiocytes, and often-detected pigmented cells have been reported to exist in the round window membrane. While the frequency with which pigmented cells are seen is said to be 9% [*Link*, 1942], they are detected quite frequently in observations of the round window membrane by a surgical microscope. These pigmented cells exist substantially in the circumference of the membrane, which corresponds to the result of *Link's* observation. It should be noted, though, that pigmented cells also exist in the round window niche. They exist only in humans, and not in other animals.

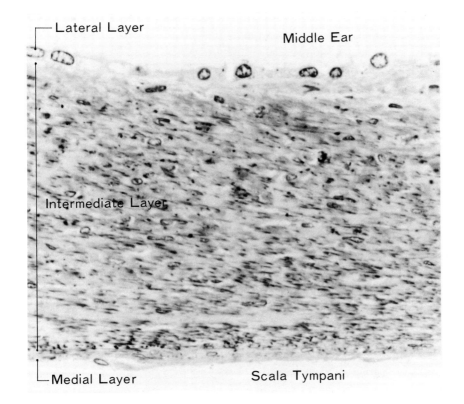

Fig. 29. Section of the human round window membrane.

These pigments lose their colors by bleaching, and the Fontana reaction test shows clearly that they are melanins. The ultrastructure of these pigmented cells will be discussed in the following section.

Transmission Electron Microscopic Findings

There have been many recent reports on the round window membrane which was observed under a transmission electron microscope. The majority are observations using round window membranes of experimental animals such as guinea pigs [*Kawabata and Paparella*, 1971; *Richardson* et al., 1971; *Arnold and Ilberg*, 1971; *Nakai and Kaneko*, 1975; *Hattori and Yuge*, 1979], dogs [*Kawabata and Ishii*, 1971], cats [*Bellucci* et al., 1972] and chinchillas

[*Paparella*, 1981]. So far, only *Hattori and Yuge* [1979] have conducted research on the round window membrane using human specimens. To understand the structure of the human round window membrane, we examined several with a transmission electron microscope.

Temporal bones of patients who died from diseases other than ear diseases were used. Immediately after temporal bones were removed, 2.5% glutaraldehyde (phosphate buffer solution pH 7.4) was injected through the tympanic membrane to the inside of the tympanic cavity. The temporal bones were fixed in the same solution for 2–3 weeks, followed by the removal of round window membranes under a surgical microscope. The round window membranes were then refixed in 1% osmic acid (phosphate buffer solution pH 7.4). They were completely dehydrated and embedded in Epon 812. Ultrathin sections were prepared and were observed under a transmission electron microscope after having been stained with uranyl acetate and lead. A human round window membrane consists of three layers extending from the middle ear to the inner ear: the outer layer, the middle layer and the inner layer. Its basic structure is the same as that of various experimental animals previously reported.

Outer Layer
Epithelial Layer (fig. 30)

The epithelial layer consists of epithelial cells continuous with the mucous membrane of the promontory. Although the cells composing this epithelial layer are generally cuboidal, in many cases they are flat cells extending along the epithelial surface. The nucleus is almost centrally located in the cytoplasm, and is round in shape. Numerous microvilli detected on the free surface of the epithelial cell are, in general, thin and short. Sometimes there are also flat cells without microvilli. Although the cytoplasm contains the usual cell organelles such as mitochondria, Golgi apparatus and endoplasmic reticulum, their development is not prominent. Occasionally, electron-dense round granules surrounded by a limiting membrane are seen. It is not known if these granules are secretory or not because of the absence of findings associated with secretion. However, it cannot be simply concluded that the granules are not secretory, as it was previously reported that the cells of the middle ear mucous membrane are potentially secretory [*Lim*, 1974]. There have been reports that some epithelial cells are ciliated cells, and ciliated cells were detected in the present study as well (fig. 34).

Basal cells existing between the epithelial cells and the basement membrane immediately beneath them are smaller and fewer than the epithelial

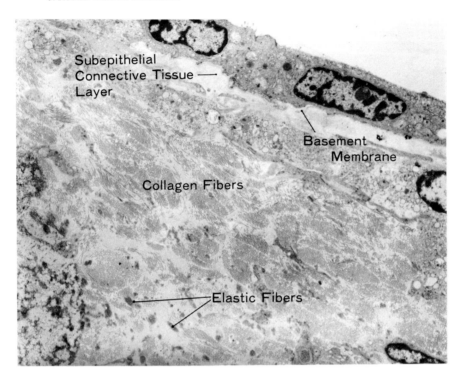

Fig. 30. The outer and middle layers of the human round window membrane (transmission electron microscopic study). × 3,000.

cells. They are irregularly polygonal in shape, and are seen clinging to the basement membrane. The nucleus of this basal cell is centrally located in the cytoplasm. This cell contains few, if any, cell organelles such as mitochondria, Golgi apparatus and endoplasmic reticulum. It is thought that the function of the basal cells in the respiratory epithelium is to supplement the epithelial cells: the basal cells in the round window membrane are thought to have more or less the same function.

Subepithelial Connective Tissue Layer

The blood vessels and nerve fibers in the round window membrane are often observed between the basement membrane immediately beneath the epithelial cells of the epithelial layer, and in the middle layer. Even when there is a lack of blood vessels or nerve fibers, the area between the basement membrane and the middle layer does not show the cellular and fibrous com-

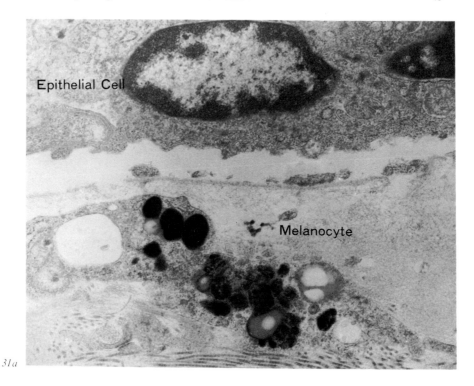

31a

ponents as tightly coexisting as they are in the middle layer: these components are, in general, scanty in this area. Furthermore, in cases of serous otitis media, for example, wandering cells seem to appear originally in this area. It is therefore believed that a subepithelial connective tissue layer lies between the epithelial layer and the middle layer.

In the present study of human round window membranes, melanocytes were detected in this area (fig. 31a, b). These cells lie in the subepithelial connective tissue layer. The melanocyte is round or oval in shape with a nucleus centrally located in the cytoplasm. This cell is characterized by the presence of many electron-dense granules surrounded by a limiting membrane in addition to the usual cell organelles. Some granules are not homogeneous substances but melanosomes showing fibrillar structures.

Middle Layer (fig. 32)

The middle layer lies between the subepithelial connective tissue layer and the inner layer, and occupies the majority of the round window mem-

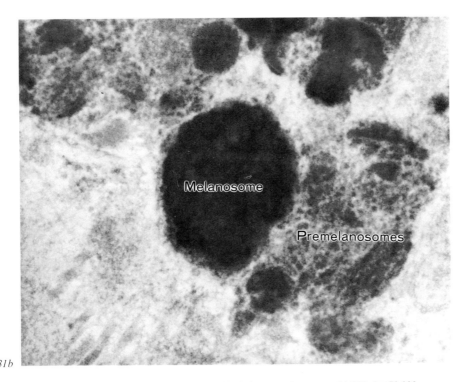

31b

Fig. 31. Melanocytes in the human round window membrane. $a \times 14{,}000$; $b \times 70{,}000$.

brane. This layer is a connective tissue layer consisting mainly of fibroblasts, collagen fibers and elastic fibers. The collagen fibers are distributed throughout this layer. Some of the collagen fibers are gathered and show the order of fiber bundles. There are, however, no apparent formations of fiber bundles, as seen in the tympanic membrane. Each collagen fiber is almost round in shape with a diameter of approximately 300–500 Å in its cross section: its vertical section, at the same time, shows a striped structure approximately 640 Å wide. It is believed, therefore, that the collagen fibers seen in the round window membrane are of the same kind as those seen in other parts of a human body. There are numerous fibroblasts existing between the collagen fibers. Generally, in cross sections of collagen fibers, fibroblasts show small cell bodies: in contrast, in vertical sections, they often show long, thin cell bodies. The fibroblast has few cell organelles.

Elastic fibers contain two components, an amorphous substance located in the central area and peripheral fibrils surrounding the center. The central

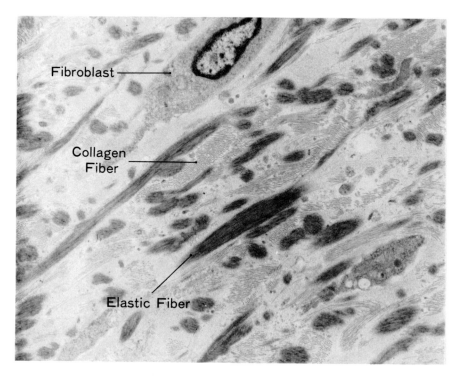

Fig. 32. The middle layer of the human round window membrane. × 6,000.

area is stained with uranyl acetate to moderate electron density. A belt of elastic fibers, of substantial length, transverses the middle layer. Elastic fibers in the middle layer usually lie in relatively larger quantities nearer the inner layer.

The morphological relation between elastic fibers and fibroblasts resembles the already-mentioned relation between collagen fibers and fibroblasts. Therefore, it is believed that elastic fibers, collagen fibers as well as fibroblasts, run in the middle layer of the human round window membrane in approximately the same direction as *Kawabata and Ishii* [1971] reported.

Inner Layer (fig. 33)

The inner layer is a continuation of the mesothelial cells lining the scala tympani of the cochlea. It shows 2–3 layers of thin and flat cells overlapping each other. The cell junctions are usually loose, and desmosomes are not detected. The intercellular spaces are wide and lack connective tissue com-

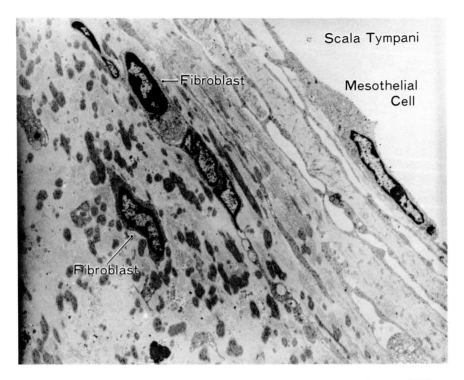

Fig. 33. The middle and inner layers of the human round window membrane. × 5,000.

ponents. Accordingly, it is easy to distinguish the inner layer from the middle layer. As mentioned above, a subepithelial connective tissue layer was detected between the epithelial layer and the middle layer, but such a connective tissue layer does not exist between the middle and the inner layers, which join directly.

Scanning Electron Microscopic Findings

For the study of the round window membrane showing its membranous structure, the scanning electron microscope study is effective because it was specifically designed to observe surface structures of specimens. In the present study, the surface structure of the human round window membrane on its middle ear side and on its inner ear side was observed, along with the structure of the connective tissue in the middle layer. The latter structure was

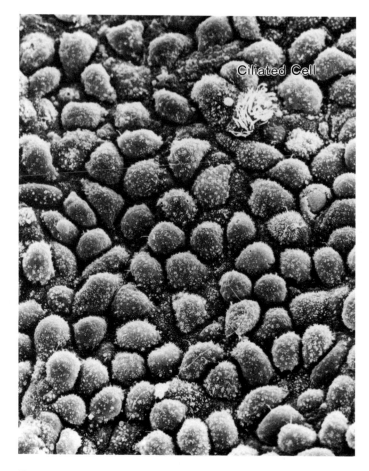

Fig. 34. The surface of the outer layer of the human round window membrane. × 1,500.

observed by peeling off the outer layer on the middle ear side, or the inner layer on the inner ear side.

Human round window membranes obtained at the time of autopsy were used. Temporal bones, immediately after the removal, were fixed in 10% formalin, and then round window membranes were collected under a surgical microscope. Some of the membranes were removed with the bony margins of the round window niches, in order to observe the running direction of the fibers in the middle layer. According to Murakami's method, the membranes were refixed in 2% tannic acid and 2% osmic acid. They were then dehydrated

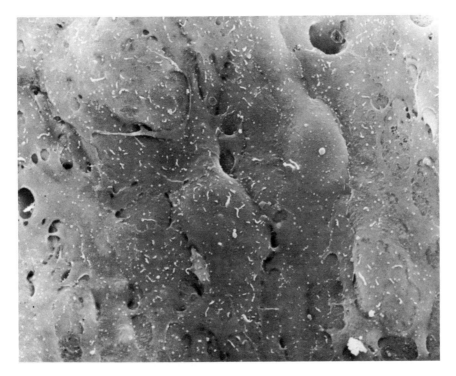

Fig. 35. The surface of the inner layer of the human round window membrane. The boundary between the cells is unclear. × 2,000.

in an ascending ethanol series, and were dried by the critical point desiccation method. Gold was evaporated onto the dried membranes by an ion spatter, and the membranes were finally studied with a scanning electron microscope. Some of the membranes, after having been fixed in 10% formalin, were transferred to a 0.5% trypsin solution (Duberco's buffer solution) to separate and dissolve the outer and the inner layers, for the purpose of observing the fibrous structure of the middle layer. The other membranes, after drying to the critical point, were placed under a stereomicroscope to peel off the outer and the inner layers, thereby exposing the middle layer.

Surface Structure of the Outer Layer (fig. 34)

The surface of the outer layer of the human round window membrane shows tight junctions of cells that are irregularly polygonal with numerous microvilli. The cells are arranged in a mosaic pattern similar to that used for paving stones. It is easy to find cell boundaries due to the terminal web formation and the slight projection of the cells as a whole towards the middle ear space, which indents the adjacent intercellular spaces. Judging from the surface structure of these epithelial cells, they are relatively large. There are few ciliated cells in the round window membrane; their surface shapes are almost identical to those of the ciliated cells seen in the middle ear space. The secretory cells with apocrine-like cellular processes on the surface were hardly detected.

Surface Structure of the Inner Layer (fig. 35)

An arrangement of large and flat cells which are irregularly polygonal in shape is seen on the surface of the inner layer. The lack of microvilli on the surface of the cells gives them a flat and smooth appearance. At times, however, part of the cell surface protrudes slightly in a dome-like shape where the nucleus of the mesothelial cell exists. The cell boundaries are often vague, as compared to the outer layer.

Observation of the Middle Layer (fig. 36)

One of the purposes of observing the middle layer of the round window membrane with a scanning electron microscope is to see the arrangement of collagen fibers and elastic fibers, the components of this layer. A study has been done on this subject using dogs [*Kawabata and Ishii,* 1971]; in the present study, the middle layer of the human round window was investigated. By removing the outer and middle layers of the round window membrane mechanically or with proteolytic enzymes, the fibrous structure of the middle layer is observable.

The fibrous structure, when observed under high magnification, is arranged mostly in bundles, rather than randomly. The bundles seem to consist of thin fibers which have merged or branched. Their form, therefore, is not as orderly as that seen in the fiber bundles in the intermediate layer of the pars tensa of the tympanic membrane [*Lim,* 1970; *Kawabata and Ishii,* 1971].

It is difficult to distinguish clearly, with a scanning electron microscope, collagen fibers from elastic fibers in the middle layer, although the two kinds of fibers were identified with a transmission electron microscope. It became clear that the fibers in the middle layer are arranged in a certain set direction, even with the human middle layer. In other words, the fibers ascend from the crista semilunaris, lying in the deep portion of the round window niche, and terminate at the opposing bony window margin. This is not to say, however,

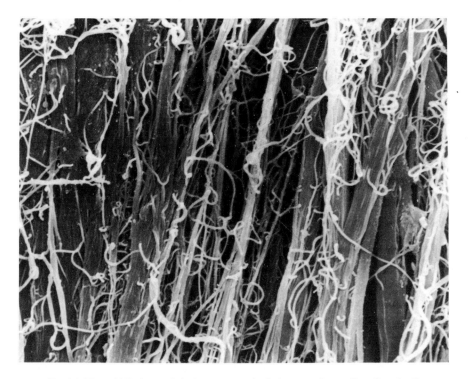

Fig. 36. The middle layer of the human round window membrane. Bundles of collagen fibers are seen. × 4,500.

that the fibers run parallel to the bony window margin. Actually, the major fiber bundles fan out slightly from the crista semilunaris to the opposing margin of the round window. The crista semilunaris is situated as though at the focal point of a fan. The basilar membrane of the hook portion inside the round window membrane is positioned approximately perpendicular to these fiber bundles.

Freeze-Fracture Method

The freeze-fracture method (freeze-cleave method, freeze-etch method) is a method of observing the ultrastructure of the tissue cells, completely different in principle from the conventional transmission electron microscopic observation method. In this method, a tissue is frozen rapidly and sec-

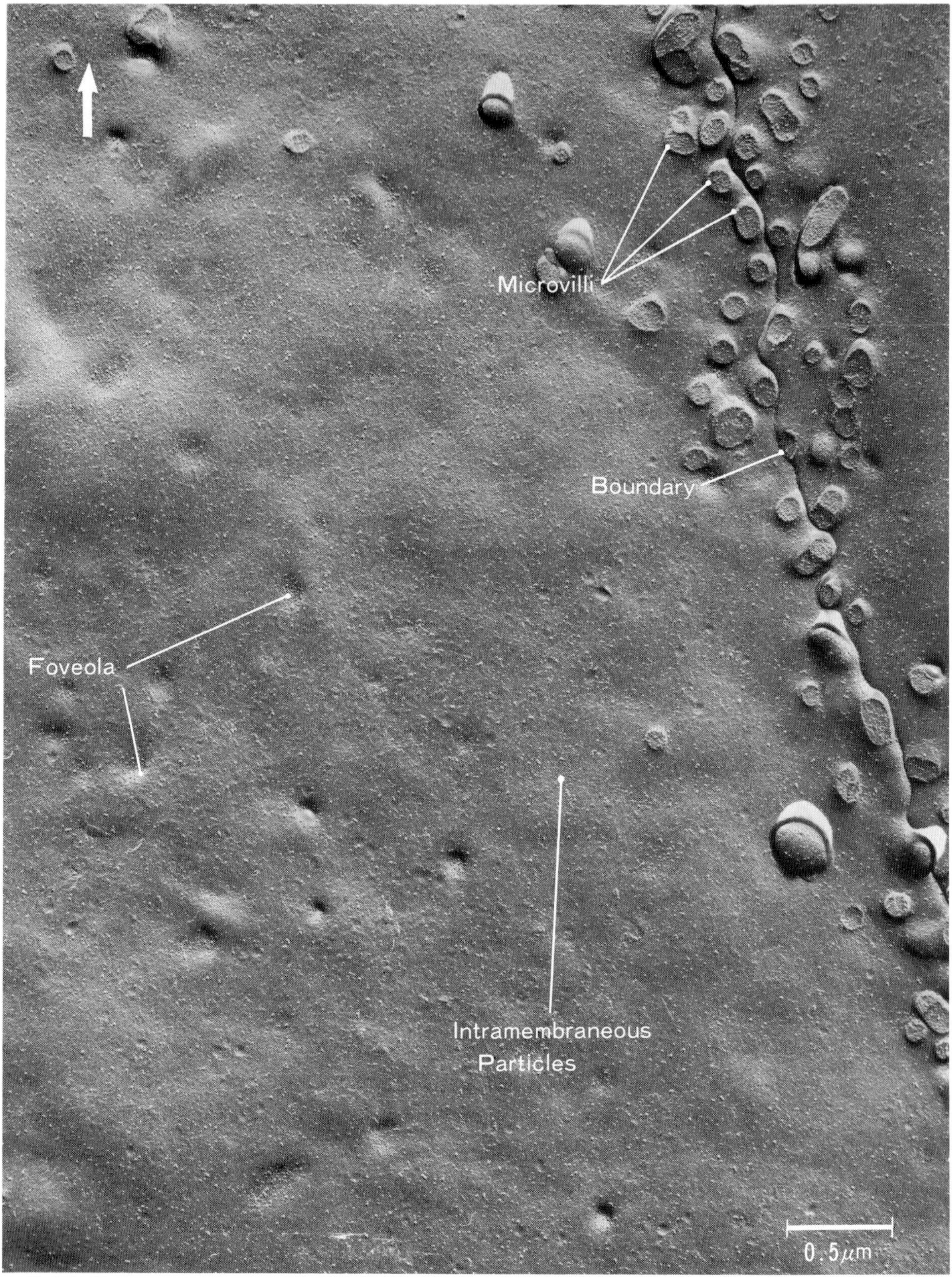

Microvilli

Boundary

Foveola

Intramembraneous
Particles

0.5 μm

tioned clearly, and platinum carbon is evaporated onto these sectioned surfaces. The membrane of each sectioned surface (replica) is observed with a transmission electron microscope. When a frozen tissue cracks, it tends to crack at the point of least resistance in terms of the tissue structure. As a cell membrane fractures along the center plane of the lipid double-layer [*Branton*, 1966], a clear view of the structure of the membrane can be obtained; moreover, it becomes clear how the ultrastructure of the cell functions differently from the cell membrane [*Staehelin*, 1974].

The junction is thought to act as a barrier that controls intercellular transmission of substances. Accordingly, the freeze-fracture method is considered useful for determining round window membrane permeability, thus observations are made on a replica of frozen sections of the round window membrane.

Albino guinea pigs of 200–300 g showing the normal Preyer's reflex were used. They were decapitated under intraperitoneal pentobarbital anesthesia. The inner ear was removed immediately after the decapitation and fixed in a mixed solution of 2.5% glutaraldehyde and 2% paraformaldehyde (0.1 *M* sodium cacodylate pH 7.4). The round window membrane was removed under a stereomicroscope while in the fixation solution, and was then dipped into a 30% glycerin solution. The round window membrane was rapidly frozen on an experiment table by Freon 22, which had been cooled by liquid nitrogen. The cutting of the membrane and the evaporating of platinum carbon were executed with a freeze-fracture apparatus manufactured by Bendix-Balzer. The replica of the membrane was prepared and then observed with a transmission electron microscope.

The round window membrane consists of the outer layer on the middle ear side, the inner layer on the inner ear side, and a middle layer located between the other two layers. The outer layer is a continuation of the mucoperiosteum of the promontory, and consists of a single layer of cuboidal cells. The inner layer shows overlapping multiple layers of flat cells lining the scala tympani of the cochlea. The middle layer is composed of collagen fibers, elastic fibers and fibroblasts. These three-layer structures can be clearly identified in the replica of the frozen membrane section, which allows a three-dimensional observation of the round window membrane as one plane.

Fig. 37. Replica of the free surface of the epithelial cells on the middle ear side (the cell membrane, P-face). There is a scattering of numerous intramembranous particles. A number of sections of microvilli are observed along the boundary of the epithelial cells. The arrow shows the direction of shadowing (guinea pig).

The distribution of microvilli was seen clearly in the replica of the surface of the epithelial cells facing the middle ear space, through the sectional view of the microvilli. Microvilli, distributed sparsely on the cell surface, often existed in groups of several strands. Numerous strands of microvilli were seen along the margin of the free surface of the cell (fig. 37). The characteristic shapes of the epithelial cells obtained from the replica observation were round and concave. There was a space protruding in the conical shape along the cut surface E-face, while the P-face showed a concavity. Both the projection and the concavity were round and 600–800 Å in diameter.

Observation of the section of the epithelial cells in the outer layer showed that the furrow-like projections formed the reticulated structure by repeating the branching and joining on the cell membrane P-face, the part facing the middle ear space, i.e., the epithelial cell surface (apicolateral region) (fig. 38). A trough-like structure was seen on the E-face, at the opposite side. The furrow-like projections tended to run almost parallel to the surface of the epithelial cells near the middle ear space side. There were many projections in this area too. This is called 'tight junction', one of the intercellular connection modes, and was the replica of so-called zonula occludens in the junctional complex seen in the sectional view through a transmission electron microscope [*Staehelin*, 1974]. The existence of zonula occludens between the epithelial cells of the round window membrane has already been reported [*Höft*, 1969; *Arnold und Ilberg*, 1971; *Arnold*, 1971]; thus the observation of this point is confirmed.

The cell junction as seen in the epithelial cells is either tight or loose depending on the number of cells, although the tight junction of the epithelial cells varies slightly in mode depending on cell type. *Claude and Goodenough* [1973] classified tight junction modes into five categories determined by the replica: very leaky, leaky, intermediate, intermediate to tight, very tight. This observation classified many tight junctions of the epithelial cells of the round window membrane as 'intermediate to tight'. The junctions of the epithelial cells are usually considered to be tight, giving morphological proof of their function of preventing the transmission of substances between the cells. In pursuing this point, it was found that the tighter the junctions in the replica were, the less permeable cells were apt to be, and thus the more resistant to epithelial permeation. There is a report on the relation between tight junctions and permeation resistance. According to the report, in the epithelial cells in the mammalian kidney, i.e., proximal convoluted tubule, resistance to the transmission of ions was hardly detected in tight junctions consisting of only one or two strands. In the bladder epithelium, however, with six or

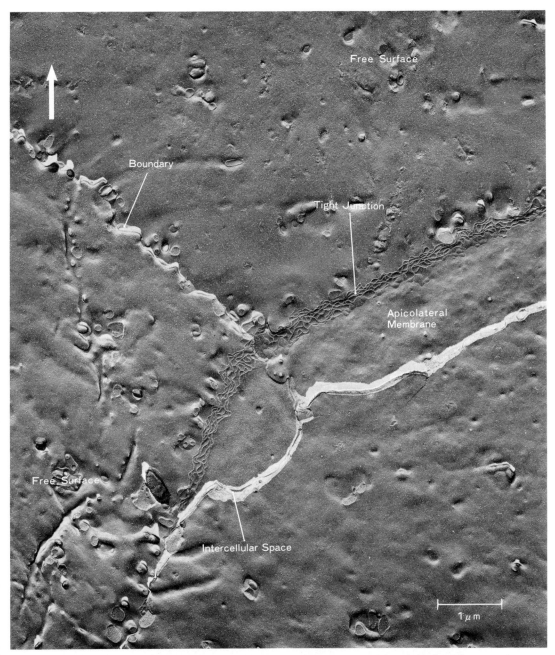

Fig. 38. Replica of the tight junction of the epithelial cells (the cell membrane, P-face). Immediately beneath the epithelial cells, numerous furrow-like projections form the reticulated structure. The arrow shows the direction of shadowing (guinea pig).

more strands, a high electric resistance existed, thereby enabling the bladder to maintain a difference in electric density with the epithelium as a boundary [*Claude and Goodenough*, 1973]. Therefore, the epithelium of the round window membrane, which had 'intermediate to tight' cell junctions, was thought to have a strong resistance to the transmission of substances. The fact that tracer experiments using thorotrast [*Höft*, 1969], ferritin [*Nakai and Kaneko*, 1975] and so on showed round window impermeability to these chemical agents could be ascribed to well-developed tight junctions of the epithelial cells in the round window membranes.

In addition to the tight cell junctions described so far, the replica of the epithelial cells occasionally shows another mode of cell junction – a slit junction (gap junction). This junction shows an orderly arrangement of small processes in the semispherical shape of approximately 90 Å in diameter on the P-face of the replica, while appearing as small foveolas in the opposing E-face [*Friend and Gilula*, 1972; *Bennett*, 1973; *McNutt and Weinstein*, 1973; *Caspar* et al., 1977]. No gap junctions in the epithelial cells of the round window membrane were detected in the present study. *Franke* [1977 a, b] also rejected the existence of gap junctions in the epithelial cells.

In the middle layer, there are few points to be clarified by observing the replica, since the cells do not assemble in this layer. However, it was noted that the replica often shows collagen fibers and elastic fibers running parallel to the sectional plane. Therefore, it is believed that replica observation would be a proper method of examining how these fibers are running.

Tight junctions were also detected in the replica of the inner layer facing the scala tympani. Specifically speaking, strand-like projections arranged in the reticulated structure were observed on the P-face of the mesothelial cells, just as they appeared in the outer layer. The E-face, on the other hand, showed trough-like concavities opposing the projections. The reticulated structure of the tight junctions was usually more irregular in the mesothelium than in the epithelium; at the same time, there were fewer junctions in the former than in the latter. As has been described before, the inner layer showed several layers of mesothelial cells, but the close contact of the whole cell body was not observed in adjacent cells. The cells had wide intercellular spaces, and they touched each other only partially. Naturally, it was where the cells were attached to each other tightly in the section specimens that tight junctions could be detected. It was not known whether tight junctions could be detected in all sites of close cell-to-cell contact. In any case, one of the functions of the tight junctions in the epithelial layer is preventing the mixing of inner ear lymph fluids and the tissue fluids of the round window membrane. Tracer experiments revealed that some substances passed from the middle ear into the inner ear through the round window membrane [*Arnold*, 1971; *Nakai and Kaneko*, 1975], which suggested that the tight junction of the mesothelial cells was not complete.

Although *Franke* [1977 a, b] has already reported the existence of gap junctions in the mesothelial cells, this cell junction mode was not observed in the present study. Named maculae communicance by *Simionescu* et al. [1975], the gap junctions are thought to provide a communication route to enable cells to have a direct mutual relationship with each other in terms of electric field and substance transmission. Since the round window membrane does not show electric excitation, the function of the gap junction, even if it exists, is unknown.

Biochemical Study of the Round Window Membrane

As described in the previous section, the round window membrane contains collagen fibers and elastic fibers. A biochemical analysis was made of the types of collagen found in the round window membrane. Human round window membranes were used as samples. At the same time, human tympanic membranes were investigated, and a comparative study was made of these membranes.

Fresh human temporal bones were removed and immediately fixed in 70% alcohol. Round window membranes and tympanic membranes were taken from the temporal bones under a surgical microscope. These samples were immersed in 100% alcohol, dehydrated, air-dried, and then weighed to determine their dry weights.

The dried tissues were then transferred to sterilized water to make them completely free of alcohol and then treated with pepsin to change insoluble collagen to soluble collagen. The pepsin solution (0.5 mg pepsin/1 ml of 0.1 M acetic acid) was filtered and sterilized. Two tympanic membranes and five round window membranes were immersed in 0.1 ml of the pepsin solution at room temperature under sterile conditions for 10 days. The pepsin solution was then freeze-dried. As a result, a white cotton-like substance (collagen pepsin) was left. The freeze-dried mixture was dissolved by heating in 0.1 ml of urea-SDS-phosphate buffer solution (8 M urea, 1% SDS, 0.05 M phosphate buffer solution pH 7.2, 0.05% bromphenol blue in 50% glycerol) at 80°C for 5 min. Under the conditions described by *Hayashi and Nagai*

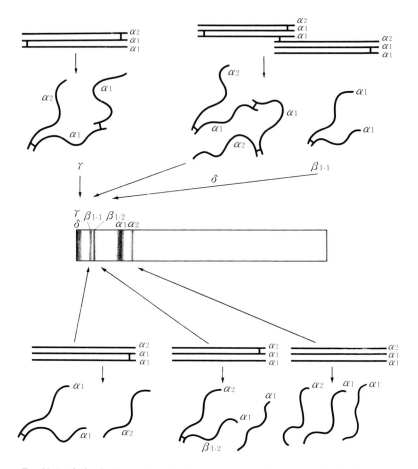

Fig. 39. Analysis of collagen. Type I collagen separates into α_1 and α_2 chains after denaturation. In molecules with a cross-link, separation does not take place and β, γ or δ chains form. These changes are identified by electrophoresis.

[1979], 50 μl of the solution obtained was subjected to SDS polyacrylamide gel electrophoresis.

When type I collagen that had been purified from cow skin by the same procedure as that described above was subjected to electrophoresis, δ, γ, β, α_1 and α_2 bands formed and traveled in the direction of electrophoretic migration. This collagen consisted of two α_1 and one α_2 chains. In molecules

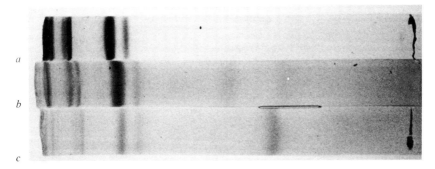

Fig. 40. Electrophoretic pattern of collagen in cow skin *(a)* and in human tympanic membrane *(b)* and round window membrane *(c).* Suspensions of human tympanic membrane and round window membrane were subjected to SDS polyacrylamide gel electrophoresis. Both membranes show the same electrophoretic pattern of collagen as seen in collagen purified from cow skin; therefore their collagens are classified as type I collagens.

which had no intramolecular cross-link, the three chains were separated from one another through denaturation by 5 min heating at 80 °C. The α_1 chain was thicker and present in larger quantities than the α_2 chain. In molecules which had an intramolecular cross-link, δ chain formed (fig. 39). The molecular weights of α_1, α_2, β and γ chains are 100,000, 100,000, 200,000 and 300,000, respectively.

Human tympanic membranes and round window membranes showed the same electrophoretic pattern of collagen as seen in type I collagen of cow skin; their collagens were classified as type I collagen by electrophoresis (fig. 40).

Permeability of the Round Window Membrane

The round window has been recognized for many years as a route through which inflammation of the middle ear spreads to the inner ear. Furthermore, it has become clear that drugs travel through the round window membrane into the inner ear. A round window membrane permeability study of various substances and drugs was carried out on animals. The following substances were used: (1) ferritin (molecular weight 445,000); (2) horseradish peroxidase (HRP) (molecular weight 40,000) and (3) triamcinolone acetonide and dexamethasone disodium phosphate, both labelled with isotopes. For substances 1 and 2, the diffusion of particles was traced with a transmission electron microscope, and for substance 3, the round window membrane permeability was investigated by measuring radioactivity in the membranous labyrinth which was dried after the administration. In addition, an experiment was conducted to investigate the migration of drugs into the inner ear fluids. Bupranolol, cefmetazole sodium, triamcinolone acetonide, and dexamethasone disodium phosphate were used.

Ferritin

Albino guinea pigs (200–300 g) showing normal middle ear mucous membrane and a normal Preyer's reflex were used in this experiment.

The tympanic bulla was clearly exposed after nembutal was injected intraperitoneally into the test animals; the round window membrane was viewed directly under a surgical microscope, while a drop of undiluted ferritin solution (Sigma Chemical Co.) was dripped with a tuberculin injector. The experimental animals were immobilized with their heads fixed in an appropriate position for 3–8 h to prevent the outflow of the undiluted ferritin solution. The middle ear space including the round window niche was then thoroughly washed with physiological saline solution. Directly after decapitation, the temporal bone was removed, fixed in 2.5% glutaraldehyde (phosphate buffer solution pH 7.4) and then refixed in 1% osmic acid. Samples obtained as controls were dehydrated in an ethanol series and embedded in Epon 812. Ultrathin sections were prepared and observed with a transmission electron microscope. Some of the sections were stained according to a special staining method [*Ainsworth and Karnovsky, 1972*] to bring out the contrast between the ferritin particles and the background; the others were stained with the usual agents such as uranyl acetate and lead.

Eustachian tube obstruction was used to induce serous otitis media in some of the guinea pigs to make a pathology group to compare with the above control group. The procedure was done in exactly the same manner on the pathology group.

Result

In controls, no ferritin particles were detected within the outer, middle and inner layers of the round window membrane. Numerous ferritin particles were seen adhering to the cell surfaces of the outer layer, but no ferritin particles were detected within the epithelial cells and in the intercellular spaces. Even 8 h after the injection of ferritin, no ferritin particles were observed in the round window membrane tissue. Therefore, it was concluded that the round window membrane did not allow ferritin particles to permeate.

Next, round window membrane permeability to ferritin particles was studied in animals with experimentally induced serous otitis media. Just after the induction, no ferritin particles were detected in the round window membrane tissue; 1–2 weeks after the induction, they were. In the outer layer, ferritin particles were detected on the cell surfaces and within the intracellular small vacuole surrounded by the membranous system but not in the intercellular spaces between the epithelial cells. In the middle layer, they existed in the spaces between collagen fibers, elastic fibers and fibroblasts; however, it did not seem that the fibroblasts contained any. In the inner layer, they were detected mainly in the mesothelial intercellular spaces, and some in the small vacuoles surrounded by the membranous system of the mesothelial cytoplasm. Thus, the animals showed ferritin particle passage at a late stage of experimentally induced serous otitis media. Moreover, these animals showed pathological changes in the round window membrane: degeneration of the epithelial cells, invasion of numerous wandering cells into the subepithelial connective tissue layer, and fragmentation of the mesothelial cell membrane in the inner layer.

Horseradish Peroxidase

The round window membrane was exposed in the same manner as in the experiment using ferritin, and a drop of 5% HRP was dripped. 2 h after that, the middle ear space was thoroughly washed with phosphate buffer solution (0.2 M pH 7.4). After decapitation, the temporal bone was removed and fixed in 2.5% glutaraldehyde for approximately 10 min. Samples were tested for HRP reaction according to the method of Graham and Karnovsky. They were then refixed in 1% osmic acid, and sections were prepared for electron microscopic observation.

Result

HRP reaction substances were detected in the round window membranes of both controls and animals with experimentally induced serous otitis media. In other words, HRP reaction substances were present in all layers: outer, middle and inner. In the outer layer, the reaction substances existed as high electron deposits on the cell surface as well as in the small intracellular vacuole surrounded by the membranous system, yet the existence of the reaction substances was not evident in the intercellular spaces between the epithelial cells. It is usually difficult to identify HRP reaction substances in the intercellular spaces between the epithelial cells where degeneration occurs during the detection procedure. HRP reaction substances were also detected in the cell body of wandering cells that had invaded into the epithelial connective tissue layer. In the middle layer, HRP reaction substances either scattered or assembled, to present an island shape or occasionally to surround the fibers, in the intercellular spaces between collagen fibers, elastic fibers and fibroblasts. In the inner layer, the mesothelial intercellular spaces and cytoplasmic vacuoles showed the existence of HRP reaction substances. These were common findings observed in both controls and animals with experimental otitis media. It was not possible to compare the amount of passage in each group.

Steroids

Tritium-labelled triamcinolone acetonide and dexamethasone disodium phosphate were used to study the round window membrane permeability. A drop of the solution was dripped onto the round window membrane, which was then left for 3 h. The middle ear space was thoroughly washed with physiological saline solution. After decapitation, the temporal bone was removed and freeze-dried immediately. In other words, the whole temporal bone was cooled in liquid nitrogen, placed in hexane and dried in a vacuum ($-60\,°C$, 10^{-4} Torr) for about 48 h, using a vacuum freeze-drying device (Type OTD-ISF, Oka Science Co., Ltd.). The auditory ossicle and the middle ear mucous membrane were completely removed from the dried sample under a stereomicroscope, and the membranous labyrinth was sampled by cracking the bony labyrinth. The sample was then divided into three groups: lower turns (basal turn and the second turn), upper turns (the third and fourth turns) and vestibule (utricle and saccule). Since the sampled tissue amounts varied in different temporal bones, the weights of the membranous labyrinths in each group were measured with a microanalyzer before the radioactivity measurement. Radioactivity counts were indicated as weight ratios.

A measurement was made of the amount of radioactive steroid placed on the round window membrane and the amount which passed into the labyrinth. The measurements obtained are shown in table V.

Table V.

	Triamcinolone acetonide dpm	Dexamethasone disodium phosphate, dpm	Control
Upper turns	1,500	72,900	115
Lower turns	2,217,200	1,120,100	168
Vestibule	30,200	44,100	107

The same procedure was used for the normal (control) cochlea except for the placement of steroid on the round window membrane.

Result

As radioactivity counts were much higher in the steroid groups than in the control group, it was thought that steroids easily passed through the round window membrane into the inner ear. High radioactivity levels were detected in the upper turns, though they were not as high as in the lower turns. Easy passage of steroids into the upper turns was recognized only 3 h after their placement on the round window membrane. The same result was obtained with regard to the vestibule.

Diffusion of Drugs into the Inner Ear Fluids

An experiment was conducted on the diffusion into the inner ear fluids of drugs placed on the round window, using bupranolol, cefmetazole sodium, triamcinolone acetonide and dexamethasone disodium phosphate.

Albino guinea pigs (200–300 g) showing a normal Preyer's reflex were anesthetized with nembutal. A posterior incision was made in the left ear to expose the tympanic bulla, which was then opened to expose the round window membrane. The animals were immobilized so that the round window membrane was fixed in a horizontal position.

Drugs used for the permeability study were as follows: bupranolol (β-receptor blocker, synthesized by *Kunz* in 1965; chemical name: l-tert-butylamino-3-(2-chloro-5-methylphenoxy)-2-propanol hydrochloride; molec. wt. 308.25); cefmetazole sodium (cephamycin antibiotic which is hardly metabolized in the body and is discharged as it is; chemical name: sodium 7β-cyanomethyl thioacetamide-7α-methoxy-3-[(l-methyl-lH-

Table VI.

Animal	Treated ear side µg Eq/ml	Control ear side µg Eq/ml
1	31.6	0
2	14.5	0
3	22.4	0

Table VII.

Animal	Treated ear side µg/ml	Control ear side µg/ml
1	255	0
2	406	13
3	224	0

tetrazol-5-yl)thio]methyl-3-cephem-4-carboxylate;   molec.   wt.   493.51); dexamethasone disodium phosphate (aqueous corticosteroid; chemical name: sodium, 9α-fluoro-16α-methylprednisolone-21-phosphate; molec. wt. 516.42); and triamcinolone acetonide (lipophilic corticosteroid; chemical name: 9α-fluoro-16α-hydroxyprednisolone acetonide; molec. wt. 434.49).

Administration
The above drugs were administered in the following ways:

Bupranolol. Bupranolol labelled with ^{14}C at the propyl position was used. Its specific radioactivity was 4.73 µCi/mg and radiochemical purity was more than 98.8%. A small piece of gelfoam soaked with 2 µl of 0.5% bupranolol solution was carefully placed on the round window membrane so as not to contact the middle ear mucous membrane. After 30 min, the round window and middle ear space were washed with 20 ml of physiological saline solution.

Cefmetazole Sodium. A small amount of gelfoam was soaked with 2 µl of 100 mg/ml cefmetazole sodium and placed on the round window membrane for 15 min. The round window and the middle ear space were then washed with 20 ml of physiological saline solution.

Dexamethasone Disodium Phosphate. 2 μl of 5 mg/ml dexamethasone disodium phosphate was placed directly on the round window membrane and left for 15 min. The middle ear was then washed with 20 ml of physiological saline solution.

Triamcinolone Acetonide. 2 μl of 10 mg/ml triamcinolone acetonide was placed directly on the round window membrane and left for 15 min. The middle ear was then washed with 20 ml of physiological saline solution.

Sampling of the Inner Ear Fluids

After the washing of the middle ear mucous membrane with physiological saline solution, the stapes was removed, and inner ear fluids were sampled from the oval window by the use of four 0.5-μl micropipettes (Drummond Scientific Co.). The sampling was done by capillarity. 2 μl of inner ear fluids in total was obtained. The procedure was done in exactly the same manner on the right (control) side, and 2 μl of inner ear fluids was obtained as a control.

Measurement of Drug Concentration

Bupranolol. The 2 μl of collected inner ear fluids was transferred to a vial and a small amount of water was added. Xylene emulsified scintillator (Amerham ACS II) was then added and mixed, and the total radioactivity was counted using a liquid scintillation counter (Beckman, Model LS-9000 system). Quenching corrections were made by the H number method using an external standard. Radioactivity was indicated as μg bupranolol equivalent (table VI).

Cefmetazole Sodium. After the addition of 50 μl of barbital solution (250 μg/ml methanol) as an internal standard to 2 μl of collected inner ear fluids, the mixture was kept in an ice bath for 10 min and centrifuged at 4°. The supernatant was subjected to high performance liquid chromatography according to the method of *Sekine* et al. [1982] for assay of cefmetazole. The operating conditions were as follows: column, μ-Bondapak C18; mobile phase, acetonitrile – 0.005 M citrate buffer (12:88); flow rate, 1.0 ml/min, and detection, 254 nm. The instrument was equipped with a pump 110A (Altex) and a detector type 440 (Waters Associates) (table VII).

Dexamethasone Disodium Phosphate. A solution of 50 μl of triamcinolone (2 μg/ml methanol), as an internal standard, was added to 2 μl of col-

Table VIII.

Animal	Treated ear side μg/ml	Control ear side μg/ml
1	1.56	0
2	1.04	0
3	1.30	0

Table IX.

Animal	Treated ear side μg/ml	Control ear side μg/ml
1	3.64	0
2	1.30	0
3	2.86	0
4	1.30	0

lected inner ear fluids; the drug concentration was measured by high performance liquid chromatography. The operating conditions were as follows: mobile phase, acetonitrile-water (50:50); flow rate, 1.5 ml/min; and the other conditions were the same as in the case of cefmetazole sodium (table VIII).

Triamcinolone Acetonide. The drug concentration was measured by the same method as in the case of dexamethasone except that dexamethasone solution (2 μg/ml methanol) was used as an internal standard (table IX).

Thus, the experimental results showed the passage of all these drugs through the membrane and into the inner ear fluids.

It has recently been noticed that several substances pass through the round window membrane and into the inner ear. There are confirmed reports of round window membrane permeation by dimethyltetracycline [*Breuninger and Giebel*, 1975], rhodamine [*Kaupp and Giebel*, 1980] and staphylococcal pyrogenic exotoxin [*Goycoolea* et al., 1980b]. In addition, it is known that ^{125}I-serum albumin (molec. wt. 70,000) does not pass through the normal round window membrane [*Brady* et al., 1976].

Nakai and Kaneko [1975] reported that ferritin passage did not occur in normal membranes, which agrees with the result obtained in our study. It was also confirmed that thorotrast, with a molecular weight as large as ferritin (445,000), did not pass through the round window membrane [*Höft*, 1968]. However, in membranes with experimental serous otitis media, ferritin passage did occur. This could be associated with degeneration of the epithelial layer. It was also reported that ^{125}I-serum albumin passed through pathologically affected membranes [*Goycoolea* et al., 1980a]. The present study confirmed that HRP invaded the round window membrane, which supports the findings of *Saijo and Kimura* [1981] and *Tanaka and Motomura* [1981].

For a round window membrane permeability study of substances with small molecular weights, substances are labelled with isotopes because their low electron density makes it difficult to carry out a tracer study with a transmission electron microscope. *Rauch* [1966] reported that ^{24}NaCl and ^{42}KCl were present in the perilymph after 1–5 min of middle ear exposure to them. Afterwards, *Brady* et al. [1976] also confirmed that relatively free passage of ^{22}Na occurred through the round window membrane. We also recognized in our study that ^{3}H-labelled triamcinolone and dexamethasone diffused from the middle ear into the inner ear.

Liquid chromatography is very useful in measuring trace amounts of drug concentration. This method allowed us to confirm that triamcinolone and dexamethasone diffused into the inner ear fluids. This time, no measurement was carried out on the amounts of drug passage into the inner ear fluids which resulted from general administration. The measured drug concentrations in the inner ear fluids were almost the same as the dexamethasone concentrations in the blood 15 min after 10 mg dexamethasone was injected intravenously into humans. This result suggested the feasibility of administering drugs via the round window as therapy for inner ear diseases if steroids rarely diffuse into the inner ear after general administration.

It was confirmed that when cefmetazole was locally used in the treatment of inner ear diseases, it readily diffused into the inner ear. In the present study, the concentration of cefmetazole, which passed through the round window membrane into the inner ear, was higher than that of the same drug in blood 10 min after 1 g cefmetazole was injected intravenously. Antibiotics do not readily diffuse into the spinal fluid, and this is thought to be true also of the inner ear fluids. The MIC of cefmetazole sodium against *Staphylococcus aureus* (FDA 209P JC) is 0.78 µg/ml. Accordingly, it can be assumed that drugs administered via the middle ear will diffuse into the cochlea to main-

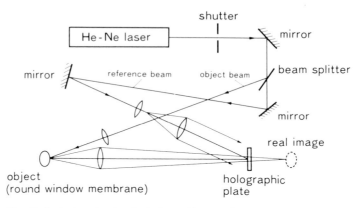

Fig. 41. Optical mechanism for holographic recording.

tain an effective drug concentration in the inner ear fluids in patients with labyrinthitis attributed to otitis media.

Bupranolol has attracted attention as a new therapeutic drug for glaucoma, and it is also used as a collyrium. If β-receptors are found to be part of the cause of Ménière's disease, the feasibility of using bupranolol to treat this disease will also be studied.

Ototoxic drugs occasionally cause severe sensorineural hearing loss, which is thought to be due to drug permeation through the round window membrane. I will refer to this again in chapter 8.

Vibration of the Round Window Membrane

The vibration pattern of the round window membrane was determined in cats by time-averaged holography for the purpose of finding the specificity of the round window membrane's vibration. Physical specificities of the round window membrane have been determined by the volumetric probe method or other techniques since *Kobrak* [1949] conducted an investigation using an optical method. The details, however, were clarified by *Khanna and Tonndorf's* [1971] time-averaged holography.

Fig. 42. a, b. Fringe order and vibration amplitude seen in the round window membrane. The frequency of the test sounds was 3,000 Hz, and a sound pressure of up to 155 dB SPL was applied. D = Dark (cat).

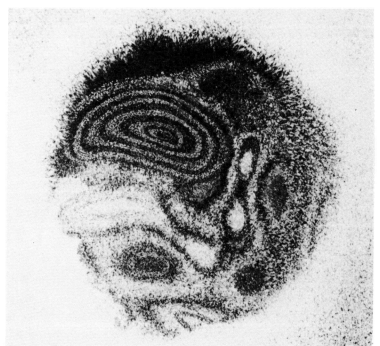

42a

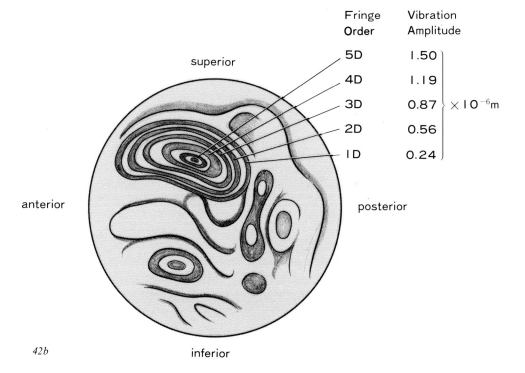

	Fringe Order	Vibration Amplitude	
	5D	1.50	
	4D	1.19	
	3D	0.87	$\times 10^{-6}$m
	2D	0.56	
	1D	0.24	

superior

anterior

posterior

inferior

42b

The present experiment was conducted to identify the specificity of the round window membrane's vibration, and the middle and the inner ears were investigated synthetically by transmitting vibrations via the external auditory meatus. In the present experiment, a cat weighing 3 kg was used under nembutal anesthesia, and five fresh cat temporal bones were also used. Vibrations were produced by a sound stimulator (Dana Japan DA-502) and transmitted via an amplifier (A-5, Yamaha) to a horn speaker. The transmitted vibrations drove the horn speaker, which then conveyed the vibrations, via tube, to the external auditory meatus. A He-Ne laser (output 25 mW) was used, and the time-averaged holography was as described in detail by *Ogura* [1974] and *Ogura* et al. [1974, 1976] (fig. 41). The frequency of the test sounds was 500–6,000 Hz, and a sound pressure of up to 155 dB SPL was applied.

Result

Both the round window membrane of the anesthetized cat and the removed temporal bones showed the most evident response at 1,500–3,000 Hz as well as marked response at low levels of sound pressure. The site that was most susceptible to vibration in response to experimentally applied vibrations was the anterosuperior portion of the round window membrane, although the amount of vibration varied greatly in individual membranes. The vibration pattern of the round window membrane was constant according to the vibration frequency of the test sound, and its pattern was simpler at lower frequencies of sound. The site of vibration was the anterosuperior portion of the round window membrane, and its vibration pattern was more complicated at higher frequencies. Change in the sound pressure did not cause any alteration in vibration patterns but increased the number of interference fringes, i.e., the vibration amplitude (fig. 42a, b).

Unlike *Khanna and Tonndorf's* [1971] experiment, the present experiment was conducted to investigate the overall response of the middle and inner ear to vibrations. Therefore, it was not possible to calculate the impedance of the inner ear, but the results suggest that the lowest impedance is at 1,500–3,000 Hz.

6. Pathology

Inflammation

It should be noted that pathology of the round window niche or the round window membrane in a human temporal bone specimen is relatively rare. The most frequently reported pathology is suppurative otitis media spread to the inner ear. There are few clinical cases of such otitis nowadays; however, the round window niche is often plagued by otitis media, or has recovered from it. In the case shown in figure 43, dense connective tissue was seen running from the round window membrane to the niche. Cell infiltration was not detected, inflammation had already subsided, and dilated capillary vessels and a large number of melanocytes as well as epithelial inclusion, in which epithelial cells were circumscribed, were observed.

Another type of case was also reported, in which labyrinthitis caused an inflammation of the middle ear through the round window membrane. Specifically, meningitis was reported to have caused an inflammation of the basal turn from the cochlear aqueduct or the modiolus through the perineural and perivascular tissues. As a result, pathological findings such as edema accompanied by bleeding and infiltration of polynuclear leukocytes were seen, localized in the round window niche or the round window membrane [Saito et al., 1981]. Serous and suppurative otitis media were induced experimentally in order to observe changes in the round window membrane under an electron microscope.

For the experiment with serous otitis media, albino guinea pigs (200–300 g) showing normal findings of the tympanic membrane and normal Preyer's reflex were used. Two methods were employed to cause serous otitis media: insertion of silicone into the pharyngeal orifice of the Eustachian tube, or opening of the tympanic bulla and corrosion of the tympanic orifice of the tube with 10% silver nitrate solution. After the above experiment, the tympanic bulla was opened up at the initial stage (on the 3rd or 4th day) and again at the late stage (at 1–2 weeks after the experiment). Upon confirmation of the retention of the fluid and the existence of edema of the mucous

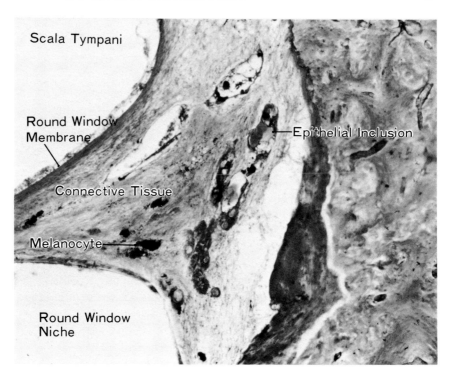

Fig. 43. Pathology of the round window niche. Male, 67 years old. Thick scar tissue adheres to the round window membrane. A large number of melanocytes and an epithelial inclusion are recognized.

membrane within the middle ear space, it was judged that serous otitis media had been experimentally induced. Guinea pigs which showed pus or reddened or swollen mucous membrane in the tympanic bulla were eliminated on the grounds of having microbial infections. An explanation of the procedure for preparing specimens is omitted in this chapter since it has been dealt with in a section of chapter 5.

Fig. 44. Normal round window membrane *(a)* and round window membrane in the early stage of experimentally induced serous otitis media *(b)*. The middle layer is edematous, and collagen fibers, elastic fibers and fibroblasts are dissociated. × 4,500 (guinea pig).

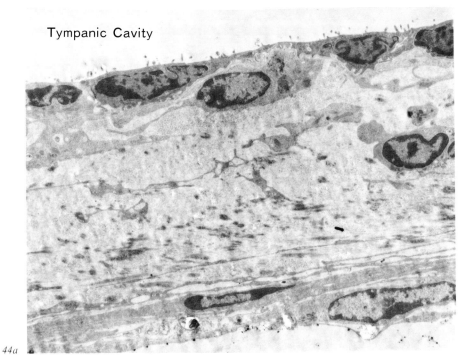

Tympanic Cavity

44a

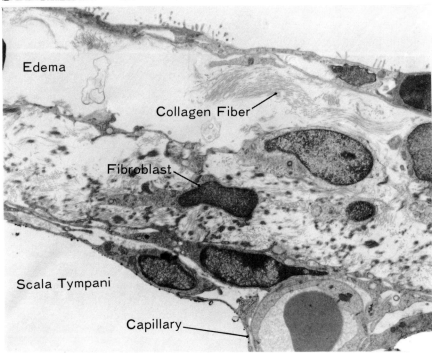

Edema

Collagen Fiber

Fibroblast

Scala Tympani

Capillary

44b

I have already described the finding of the normal round window membrane obtained from a transmission electron microscopic study. In early-stage serous otitis media, major changes occur in the middle layer. The entire middle layer becomes edematous; furthermore, the collagen fibers, elastic fibers and fibroblasts which are closely aggregated in the normal condition become dissociated and show a loose arrangement (fig. 44a, b). However, the present study showed no significant changes in the collagen fibers, elastic fibers or fibroblasts. In the outer layer, neither degeneration nor sloughing off of cells was observed, and there was no change in the structure of the basement membrane. Also in the inner layer, two or three layers of flat cells were seen in the overlapped form, which was almost the same as in the normal membrane.

In the late-stage observation, after 1–2 weeks, there were more prominent changes in the round window. In the middle layer, the edematous condition progressed further, and it seemed as if the collagen fibers, elastic fibers and fibroblasts were existing independently. However, these minute structures themselves did not show any notable changes. In the outer layer, the electron density of the cytoplasm became higher in some of the epithelial cells. It also became difficult to distinguish among organelles such as mitochondria, Golgi apparatus and endoplasmic reticulum; there were changes that could be associated with the early stage of cell degeneration. In the subepithelial connective tissue layer, wandering cells such as polymorphonuclear leukocytes were often detected. Wandering cells are rarely seen in the middle or the inner layer, and they do not seem to wander much into the middle ear through the outer layer either. These wandering cells were thought to have originated from the capillary vessels existing in this layer. However, the minute structure of the vessels did not show any significant changes. The inner layer did not show any pathology suggesting degeneration of the mesothelium. Instead, numerous granular particles of high electron density and of varying size were often seen adhering to the surface of the cells facing the scala tympani. While it is interesting to note that such granular particles appear on the surface of the mesothelial cells of the round window membrane in ears with experimentally induced serous otitis media, their characteristics or functions have not been clarified yet.

Next, in order to induce experimentally suppurative otitis media, 0.3–0.5 ml of a suspension of *Staphylococcus aureus* 209p strain in physiological saline solution (number of bacteria 9×10^6/ml) was injected into the tympanic bulla of albino guinea pigs through the tympanic membrane using a tuberculin injector.

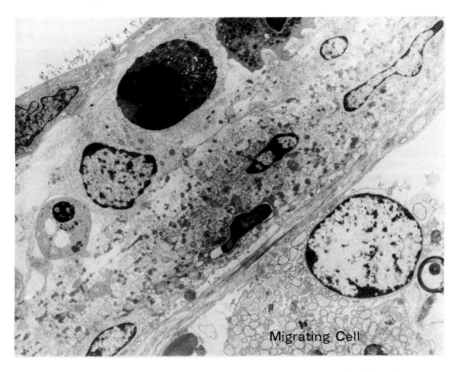

Migrating Cell

Fig. 45. Pathology of the round window membrane in experimentally-induced suppurative otitis media. × 4,500 (guinea pig).

24 h after the injection, the guinea pigs were decapitated. The tympanic bulla showed serous secretion, and the mucous membrane was reddened and swollen. The outer layer surface of the round window membrane showed a large amount of fine precipitate, and there was little sloughing off or degeneration of the epithelial cells. The middle layer showed marked edema with bleeding and polymorphonuclear leukocyte infiltration, but no significant change in arrangement of fibers was noted. In the inner layer, no major change was detected, but the scala tympani facing the round window membrane showed bleeding with wandering cells (fig. 45). After 72 h, the animals' tympanic bullae were entirely filled with bleeding granulation. The round window membrane also showed formation of the granulation tissue.

Otosclerosis

It is well known that otosclerosis occurs mostly in the anterior portion of the oval window, and that conductive hearing loss will occur if the annular ligament is invaded. However, a study of human temporal bone specimens showed that only a small fraction of patients with a focus of otosclerosis revealed clinical symptoms. As there are many patients who do not show any clinical symptoms, the existence of otosclerosis cannot be confirmed in these cases until a histological examination is conducted after death [*Guild,* 1944]. An examination of such histological otosclerosis in temporal bone specimens showed that a round window focus was present in approximately 40% of ears examined [*Nylén,* 1949]. Although it is thought that a focus in this area does not usually cause any clinical symptoms, hearing loss will occur if the focus becomes large enough to close off the round window niche. Moreover, in this area, the focus often invades the endosteal layer, even in the early stage of the lesion, resulting in protrusion into the scala tympani [*Fleischer,* 1962]. When the endosteal layer is invaded extensively, sensorineural hearing loss occurs [*Lindsay,* 1973].

We also examined a patient with histological otosclerosis who had a focus in the round window. The following is our report on this case [*Harada* et al., 1975]:

Male subject, 82 years old. Died from pneumonia. In the audiogram taken almost a year before death, the left ear showed mixed type hearing loss at approximately 50 dB. The patient had been suffering from hearing loss in the right ear ever since head trauma which occurred during the war.

Findings of the left temporal bone (fig. 46): Otosclerotic foci were detected in three areas of the bony labyrinth. The most active focus was in the promontory adjacent to the round window. This focus invaded the endosteal layer, and part of it protruded into the scala tympani. However, neither atrophy of the spiral ligament nor invasion to the round window membrane was detected. The other two foci were seen in the anterior wall of the internal auditory meatus and in the anterolateral portion of the bony labyrinth. A marked excavation in the posterosuperior portion of the tympanic membrane led us to guess that conductive loss, a component of mixed-type hearing loss in this case, was caused by the pathologies of the middle ear and that sensorineural loss, the other component, was due to presbyacusis. Therefore, the hearing loss was not due to otosclerosis.

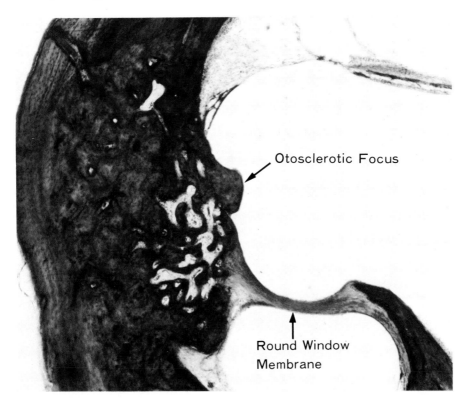

Otoslerotic Focus

Round Window
Membrane

Fig. 46. Otosclerosis: male, 82 years old. The focus partially protrudes to the scala tympani.

Tumor

There are different ways in which invasion of malignant tumors into the round window occurs: direct invasion of middle ear tumors, invasion of metastatic tumors through the internal auditory meatus, and hematogenous invasion. In each of these cases, the tumor cells can invade any tissue. The following report is of a case with cochlear lesion caused by metastatic tumor, and changes observed in the vicinity of the round window are discussed:

Male subject, 71 years old. In May 1970, a paralysis occurred on the left side of the face, followed by rapid and severe hearing loss in both ears in June. He was diagnosed as having lung cancer, and died in August.

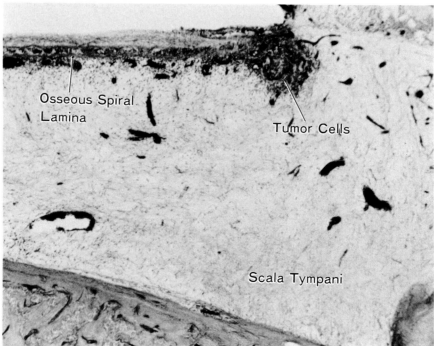

47a

Findings of the left temporal bone (fig. 47a, b): Extensive metastasis of lung cancer was noted in the meninx, and so-called leptomeningeal carcinosis occurred. Metastasis of adenocarcinoma was seen within the internal auditory meatus, and the surrounding bones were destroyed. Tumor cells had infiltrated and proliferated in the modiolus and the scala tympani of the basal turn, causing fibrosis in the surrounding tissue. The perilymphatic cavity had disappeared. Development of the capillary vessels was prominent. In part of the fibrotic scala tympani collagen fibers were grouped together, which seemed to be a sign of preossification. The fibrosis of the scala tympani was not limited to the area adjacent to the round window membrane, but was also seen in part of the round window niche.

Tumor cells were also detected in the round window niche to a slight degree. This suggests that these cells had infiltrated the middle ear side through the significantly thickened round window membrane.

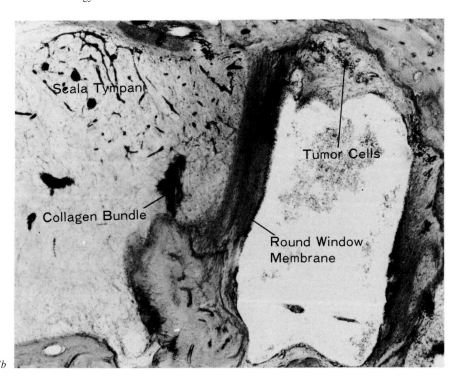

47b

Fig. 47. a, b. Metastasis of lung cancer into the internal auditory meatus. Male, 71 years old. The tumor cells have entered the scala tympani of the basal turn, and some have infiltrated into the round window niche through the significantly thickened round window membrane. The scala tympani has all but gone through complete fibrosis, and part of it shows a bundle of collagen fibers.

Disturbance of Circulation

Various pathologies are induced in the inner ear by circulatory disturbance in the region. For example, it is known that if the inner ear artery is blocked up experimentally, the cochlea will eventually become ossified [*Kimura and Perlman*, 1958]. This tendency was recognized in humans as well as animals [*Belal*, 1980].

In this section, a case of essential cryoglobulinemia which we recently examined is introduced [*Nomura* et al., 1982].

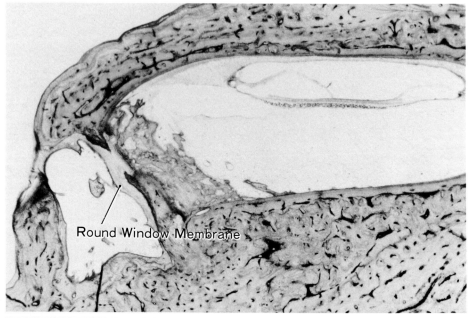

48a

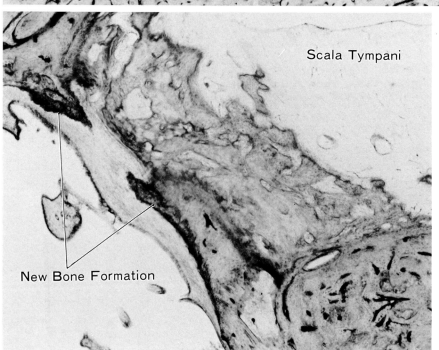

48b

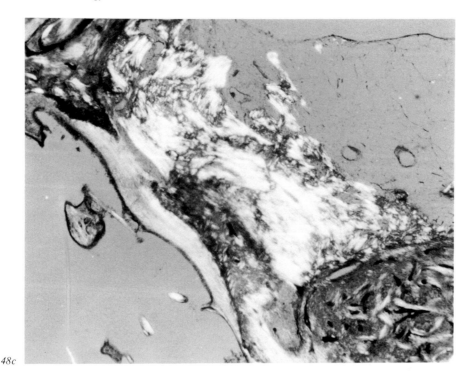

48c

Fig. 48. a–c. Cryoglobulinemia. Female, 44 years old. Ossification is seen touching the round window membrane. The round window membrane itself near the window margin shows new bone formation *(a).* The enlarged view of this new formation *(b),* when observed under a polarizing microscope, shows a laminar structure in the newly formed bone in the bony labyrinth and in the scala tympani. The new bone formation in the round window membrane does not show a laminar structure *(c).*

Female subject, 44 years old. Since 1962, petechiae, small ulcers as well as cyanoses had been appearing in the lower thighs in wintertime, but were alleviated in warmer weather. In 1972, she started having ringing in the ears, and her hearing became gradually more impaired. In 1978, a hearing test revealed that hearing loss had occurred in both ears. 1 week after the examination, she died of bronchopneumonia.

Findings of the left temporal bone (fig. 48a–c): Two major changes were observed: one was the presence of an eosinophilic precipitate within the scala media, and the other was ossification of the vestibulum and semicircular canals of the basal turn. In the cochlea, ossification was localized in the scala tympani, and fibrous tissue containing melanocytes was attached to the bone tissue. The round window membrane was thickened and a wedge-shaped formation of new bone was found protruding from its attachment area to the center of the membrane. The residual membrane was also attached to the new bone formation in the scala tympani, but the mesothelium remained in between.

A polarizing microscopic examination showed that the ossified area of the scala tympani had a laminar structure like the bony labyrinth, while the new bone formation of the round window membrane did not, indicating that pathological changes in the two areas occurred at noticeably different times. Although we could not clarify why ossification occurred in the basal turn due to circulatory disturbance, it was apparent in the present case that ossification took place first in the scala tympani and later in the round window membrane.

We also examined a case with no history of ear disease in which a temporal bone specimen showed partial ossification in the round window membrane (fig. 49).

Others

In infants, a large amount of mesenchymal tissue is present in the middle ear, including the round window niche. This tissue is gradually absorbed. In a temporal bone specimen with the Mondini-type anomaly, polyp-like tissue was seen in the round window niche (fig. 50).

An infant girl, 2 months old. Hydrocephalus was detected. Histologically, atrophy and edema were observed in the brain parenchyma. There were no major changes in the external ear or the tympanic membrane. Although the internal carotid artery protruded in the tympanic cavity, there was no abnormal change in the middle ear structure. The cochlea was 9.5 mm long on the left, 8.5 mm on the right, and on both sides, only the lower parts of the basal turns were recognized. All the factors contribute to a diagnosis of the Mondini-type anomaly [*Nomura and Hiraide*, 1972]. On the left side of the temporal bone, the mesenchymal tissue protruded, polyp-like, into the round window niche, with part of the protrusion touching the round window membrane. Incidentally, the cochlear aqueduct was significantly large, with a diameter of 380 μm.

Although the middle ear space is filled with mesenchymal tissues for a while after birth, such tissues gradually become absorbed and the space becomes covered by mucoperiosteum.

Embryologically, the round window niche is closely related to the inner ear and the cranial cavity. The fact that melanocytes which are seen frequently in the inner ear are observed in this region of the middle ear is an

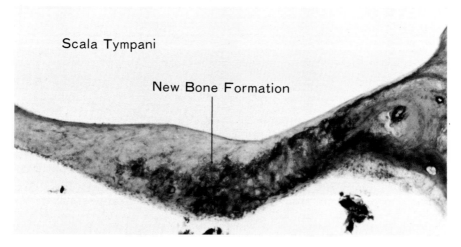

Fig. 49. Ossification of the round window membrane. Male, 67 years old.

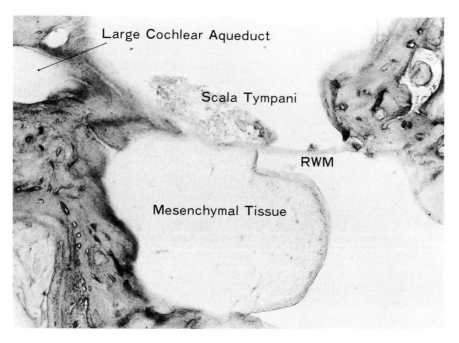

Fig. 50. Mondini-type anomaly. An infant girl, 2 months old. Mesenchymal tissue seen in the round window niche. The cochlear aqueduct is significantly wide. RWM = Round window membrane.

indication that there is a strong relationship between the inner ear and the round window niche. This region is considered to be a special area in the middle ear.

It has been reported that in the temporal bone of a patient with Down's syndrome, the round window niche showed severe stenosis and a large portion of the niche was filled with mesenchymal tissues [*Harada and Sando*, 1981].

In cases of cretinism, the promontory of the temporal bone becomes substantially hypertrophic by proliferation of bones. The niche is extremely narrow and contains adipose tissue. Hypoplasia of the round window niche is a characteristic finding in cretinism [*Nager*, 1926].

7. Anatomy of the Circumference of the Round Window

There are various structures surrounding the round window. I will describe separately those on the middle ear side and those on the inner ear side.

Structures on the Middle Ear Side

Since the round window lies posteroinferior to the tympanic cavity, it is close to the posterior tympanic wall, or the posterior aspect of the medial tympanic wall and the hypotympanum. The subiculum promontorii is a bony trabecula extending posteriorly from the posterior or superior wall of the round window niche; it forms an inferior limit of the sinus tympani. The cul-de-sac, the terminating portion of the cochlea, is located inside of the subiculum promontorii.

A large air cell can sometimes be seen extending anteroinferiorly from the round window niche (fig. 51). This air cell is the hypotympanic cell tract running towards the inferior portion of the labyrinth from the hypotympanum, and is a part of the perilabyrinthine cell tracts. Although this air cell is usually not seen during middle ear surgery, it is often seen in a tomogram of the temporal bone (fig. 52).

The jugular bulb exists under the inferior wall of the tympanic cavity. Its size and position vary. However, when the bulb is small, it is usually separated from the middle ear space by a thick bony wall. This bone is compact, but it sometimes becomes pneumatized by the air cell of the hypotympanum. When the jugular bulb is situated in a high position, it can partially enter the middle ear and become protruded. Furthermore, even when the bulb is covered by a bony wall, there are instances where it is very thin and slightly defective.

The bony wall enclosing the jugular bulb is called the dome of the jugular bulb. Although the round window niche is usually concave, a high jugular bulb dome effects curvature, making the niche extremely shallow (fig. 53).

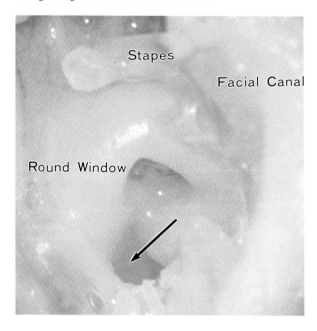

Fig. 51. The air cell surrounding the labyrinth. A large air cell is open in the round window niche (arrow).

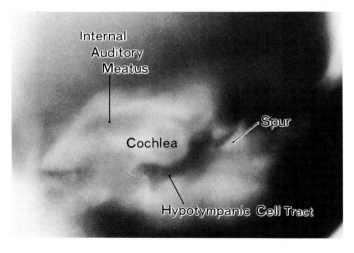

Fig. 52. A tomogram of the temporal bone. The hypotympanic cell tract opens to the round window niche.

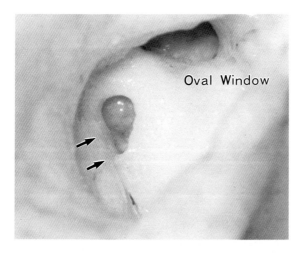

Fig. 53. The shallow round window niche. The high positioning of the jugular bulb raises the niche (arrows).

It has already been mentioned that the dome and the posterior semicircular canal are close to each other. When the dome is low, it is 3 mm below the posterior semicircular canal, but when the dome is high, it touches the ampullated end of the posterior semicircular canal. In the latter case, there is a possibility of damaging the jugular bulb when surgically removing the posterior semicircular canal, or of damaging the posterior semicircular canal when performing surgery in the vicinity of the jugular bulb [*Graham*, 1977].

The round window niche has the appearance of a small dome situated over the dome of the jugular bulb. Furthermore, the round window membrane is parallel to this structure as a whole, thereby running almost parallel to the apex of the jugular bulb. It is a coincidence of phylogenesis that these structures are in such close proximity. In the frog (*Rana*), the perilymphatic sac and the jugular bulb touch each other.

Structures on the Inner Ear Side

The lower part of the pars anterior of the round window membrane is attached to the crista semilunaris. The aperture of the cochlear aqueduct in the scala tympani is adjacent to the crista semilunaris (fig. 54). The diameter

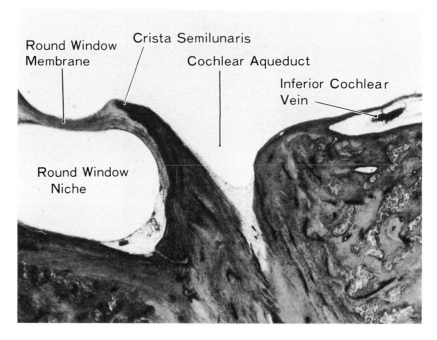

Fig. 54. The cochlear aqueduct and crista semilunaris.

of this aperture varies depending upon the site and direction in which a measurement is made; it is reported to be about 0.1 mm on average [*Anson et al.*, 1964; *Ritter and Lawrence*, 1965]. The inferior cochlear vein, which collects the venous blood of the cochlea, runs in a different bony canal from the cochlear aqueduct: the first accessory canal. The inferior cochlear vein drains either into the inferior petrosal sinus or directly into the jugular bulb. This accessory canal lies apical to the aperture of the cochlear aqueduct, with a distance between the two of 0.1–0.3 mm [*Palva and Dammert*, 1969] or 0.1–0.2 mm [*Rask-Andersen et al.*, 1977].

The cochlear aqueduct runs parallel to the internal auditory meatus in a view of the temporal bone from above. Its length is approximately 10 mm [*Meurman*, 1930; *Anson et al.*, 1965; *Rask-Andersen et al.*, 1977], although there are reports of 6.5 and 6.2 mm as well [*Ritter and Lawrence*, 1965; *Palva and Dammert*, 1969]. Our measurement was taken by dissecting the decalcified temporal bone to expose the cochlear aqueduct. The lengths of the aqueducts were 9–12 mm, with the average for the five specimens being 10 mm (fig. 55).

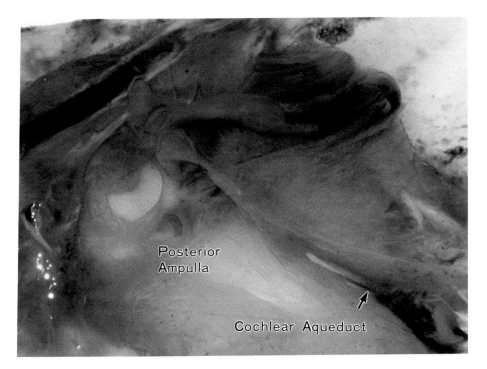

Fig. 55. The cochlear aqueduct.

The scala tympani is on the inside of the round window membrane. The round window membrane is situated lateroinferiorly with respect to the scala tympani close to its end, not at the end of the scala tympani. In other words, the scala tympani lies superior to the round window membrane and not anterior to it. The terminating point of the scala tympani (cul-de-sac) lies slightly posterior to the pars posterior of the round window membrane. As mentioned before, the lower part of the pars posterior is attached to the osseous spiral lamina. In a section view of this part of the cochlea, the scala tympani is triangular, while the pars anterior is wider and almost circular.

After the dissection of the temporal bone from the tegmen to enter the vestibule, the osseous spiral lamina and its surroundings can be observed. This observation shows that there is a deep bony depression touching upon the terminating portion of the osseous spiral lamina. This is the posterior ampulla, containing the ampullated posterior semicircular canal (fig. 56). From the middle ear side, the bulge of the bone corresponding to this ampulla is indistinct.

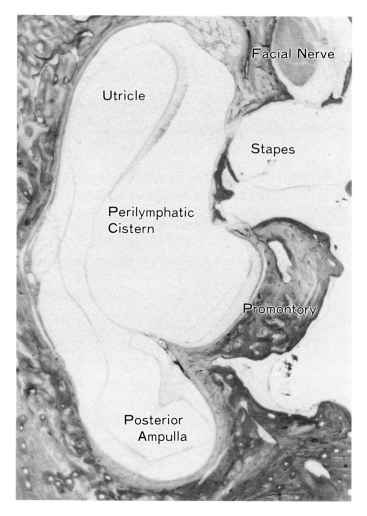

Fig. 56. Vertical section of the vestibule.

The part of the vestibular organs that is the closest to the round window niche is the ampulla of the posterior semicircular canal. The nerve of the posterior ampulla is also called the singular nerve, and it has 2,780–3,500 myelinated nerve fibers [*Bergström,* 1973]. The singular nerve ramifies from the inferior division of the vestibular nerve in the internal auditory meatus and runs through a small duct, the singular canal, which originates in the meatus. *Gacek's* [1961] observation that the singular nerve has small branches was

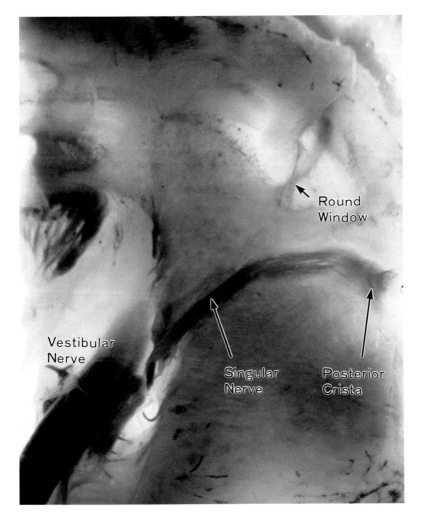

Fig. 57. The singular nerve.

confirmed in all of 640 temporal bones observed by *Montandon* et al. [1970] and in 78% of 223 temporal bones examined by *Okano* et al. [1980].

The singular canal does not run linearly. The singular nerve runs almost parallel to the internal auditory meatus to the outside; but at the same time it curves posteriorly immediately below the vestibule to connect with the ampulla of the posterior semicircular canal (fig. 57). The length of the singular canal was approximately 7 mm on average for five specimens.

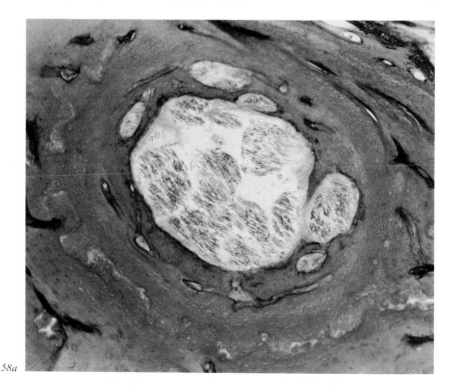

58a

Although the singular canal is a simple bony canal near the internal auditory meatus, it separates toward its end into small canalicules by bony tissue. This is apparent from a section specimen (fig. 58a, b); it also is observable with a surgical microscope in a dissected specimen that the nerve ramifies into nerve bundles at a certain point.

The singular nerve is almost parallel to the lower attachment area of the round window (the pars posterior) near the ampulla of the posterior semicircular canal. This makes the round window membrane an indicator for finding the singular nerve in singular neurectomy. The distance between the two is approximately 1 mm.

Looking at the temporal bone externally, the ampulla of the posterior semicircular canal lies posterior to the line connecting the posterior margins of the oval window and the round window [*Epley*, 1980].

Judging from vertical section specimens including the round window membrane and the oval window (fig. 59), the measurements related to the singular nerve are as follows (10 ears used): diameter of the singular nerve

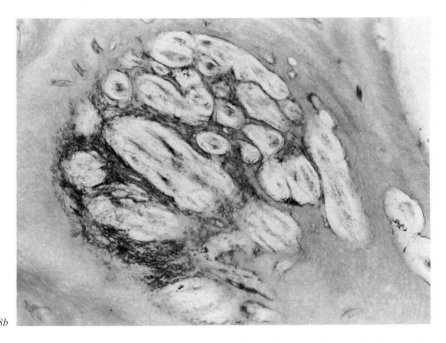

58b

Fig. 58. a, b. Sections of the singular nerve. Nearing the posterior ampulla, the singular nerve separates into bundles that run through the small bone canals. a and b are almost the same site in specimens from different patients.

(including all small nerve bundles): 0.45–0.85 mm; shortest distance between the singular nerve and the round window niche: 0.53–1.28 mm; shortest distance between the singular nerve and the medial wall of the vestibule: 0.22–0.48 mm.

Microfissure

The presence of a microfissure between the ampulla of the posterior semicircular canal and the round window niche has been known for many years, and numerous theories have been advanced about its origin. It can be seen only in tissue specimens of human temporal bones; it has not been reported in other animals or in dry skull specimens.

The microfissure exists in the area from the round window niche facing the round window membrane to the crista ampullaris of the posterior semicircular canal. It is a space in the bone, with a width of approximately

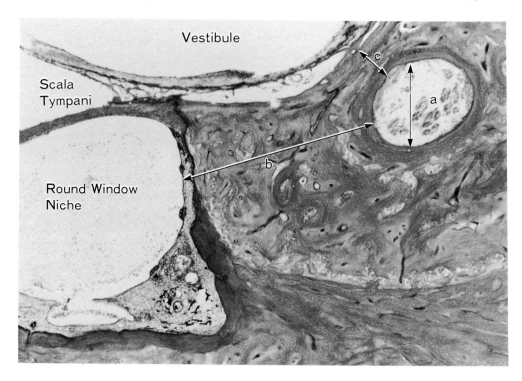

Fig. 59. Measurements pertaining to the singular nerve. a = Diameter of the nerve; b = shortest distance between the singular nerve and the round window niche; c = shortest distance between the singular nerve and the vestibule.

30–50 μm, which contains connective tissue. Figure 60 shows the microfissure in a sample specimen: both sides of the space boundary surfaces have been strongly stained with hematoxylin. The microfissure cannot be detected in a specimen taken at birth. It gradually becomes observable after the first year of age, and there is a report of its observation in all infants over 6 years of age in one study [*Okano* et al., 1977].

Although the microfissure has sometimes been discussed in relation to the development of otosclerosis, its clinical significance is unknown at present. As a route which connects the middle and inner ears, the microfissure may be responsible for the spread of inflammation and/or the occurrence of drug-induced hearing loss. A similar microfissure exists in the vicinity of the oval window [*Harada* et al., 1981].

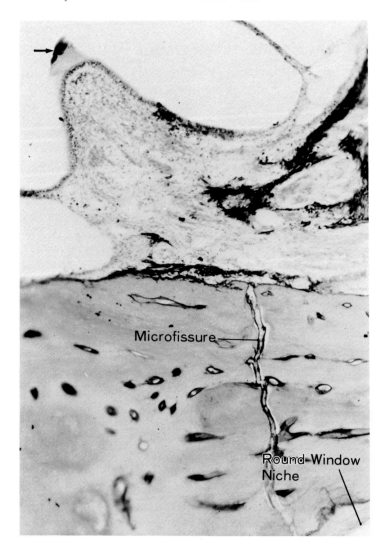

Fig. 60. Microfissure. In this case, cupulolithiasis is seen in the cupula (arrow). Both sides of the space boundary surfaces have been stained with hematoxylin.

8. Ear Diseases Pertaining to the Round Window

Drug-Induced Hearing Loss

Various diseases traceable to either the external ear or the middle ear are treated with eardrops. In order to inhibit the growth of bacteria and mold, the acidity of the drops is enhanced by adding boric or acetic acid. Although there have been reports on the influence of changes in pH on the round window membrane, drug-induced hearing losses, as described in this section, are often detected when eardrops containing ototoxic antibiotics are used. These hearing losses are due to the ototoxic antibiotics entering the cochlea from the middle ear.

Most antibiotics used as eardrops are ototoxic drugs such as fradiomycin (neomycin) and chloramphenicol. Polymyxin was used at one time. Fradiomycin is effective against gram-negative bacilli such as coliform bacillus, while polymyxin E, otherwise known as colistin, kills gram-negative bacilli, especially *Bacillus pyocyaneus,* coliform bacillus, Klebsiella and Enterobacteriaceae. These drugs, therefore, were used either separately or in combination. Drugs used as eardrops must: (1) have a wide antibacterial spectrum; (2) have few resistant bacteria; (3) be stable to chemicals, pH and heat; (4) not be inactivated by blood and/or secretions; (5) exert little local action, and (6) not become antigenic.

There are two factors to be considered in using eardrops. The first is the question of whether they can produce a satisfactory drug concentration in an affected site and, furthermore, whether such a concentration can be maintained for a certain period of time. A drug may merely cover the surface of the exudate and not penetrate deeply into the tissue. With an area as complex as the middle ear, eardrops might not even reach an inflammatory site. In such a case, not only would eardrops have no beneficial effect, but they might have the kind of harmful effects described below.

The second factor to be considered is that sensorineural hearing losses can be induced by ototoxicity. Fradiomycin, for example, is the most toxic of all ototoxic antibiotics, and, for this reason, some drug advertisements state

that fradiomycin should not be used in cases of tympanic membrane perforations.

Fradiomycin does not decompose internally, and it acts ototoxic if it
reaches the inner ear, wherever it may be absorbed from. Therefore, it is possible for it to be absorbed through the diseased skin of the external auditory
meatus even though the tympanic membrane has no perforation, and sensorineural hearing loss can be caused if a substantial quantity is absorbed.
In reality, however, most drug-induced hearing losses occur in ears that have
relatively large perforations.

In considering the possible ways eardrops can enter the cochlea, the
round window membrane is the most likely route when one considers the
anatomy of the ear itself. In patients with large perforations, which allow eardrops to easily enter the middle ear, the medial wall of the tympanic cavity
receives the drug when the affected ear faces upward. It is possible for the
drug solution to enter the round window niche in this position. If the patient
then stands, the drug solution will move to the hypotympanum; however,
some of the solution might remain in the round window niche, depending on
the quantity of the solution. In a supine position, the solution would move
towards the sinus tympani, and the round window niche would be filled with
the drug solution. Thus, the round window niche would always be exposed
to drug solutions. It goes without saying that conditions vary according to the
shape of the niche, its depth and the existence of connective tissue.

Clinical Picture of Drug-Induced Hearing Loss

Drug-induced hearing loss presents a clear clinical picture, characterized
by the following features:

(1) *Use of eardrops:* Eardrops containing ototoxic antibiotics are continuously used for a relatively long period of time, for at least 1 month. Patients
often continue using eardrops every day at their own volition.

(2) *Appearance of the tympanic membrane:* A large perforation is usually
recognized. When a perforation is small, not allowing the easy entrance of
a drug solution into the tympanic cavity, hearing loss is not caused. The state
of the tympanic cavity also affects the possibility of hearing loss, but there
are many cases where hearing loss occurs in an ear with a relatively clean and
more or less normal-looking tympanic cavity.

(3) *Audiogram:* Characteristically, drug-induced hearing losses show the
development of severe sensorineural hearing losses first in the high frequen-

cies. In other words, the audiograms first show the development of hearing loss at 8,000 Hz, and then show the progression of the hearing loss at 4,000 Hz, 2,000 Hz, and finally at all frequencies. All audiograms reveal similar tracings of severe hearing loss. The hearing loss progresses to a certain degree even after the termination of the use of eardrops, requiring up to several months before the progression stops.

This clinical picture makes the diagnosis of many cases of drug-induced hearing loss easy. It should be noted, however, that there are some cases of chronic otitis media which show lesions of the cochlea caused not by eardrops but by bacterial infection or by inflammatory products. These cases also show sensorineural hearing losses in the high frequencies [*Paparella* et al., 1970]. Therefore, it is sometimes difficult to make a definite diagnosis of drug-induced hearing loss; it would be useful in making a differentiation to observe the round window niche and the round window membrane.

Subject K.T., a 52-year-old female. For 30 years or so, the patient had been suffering from chronic otitis media in both ears, occasionally accompanied by otorrhea. The tympanic membranes in both ears had large central perforations. In 1974, the patient used an eardrop containing fradiomycin daily for 7 months. The audiograms in figure 61 for February 1974 show the hearing before the use of eardrops, while those for December 1974 show that after the medication. Although the use of eardrops was discontinued, hearing loss progressed, especially in the right ear. The audiogram scaled out at all frequencies 8 months later. The left ear was saved in frequencies other than 4,000 and 8,000 Hz. Although the patient complains of tinnitus in both ears, it is stronger in the left ear.

As preventive measures, the following should be kept in mind:

(1) There is a possibility that eardrops, particularly those containing ototoxic antibiotics, may induce sensorineural hearing losses when they are used in cases with a relatively large perforation in the tympanic membrane.

(2) Application of strong positive and negative pressure to the middle ear with a magnifying otoscope may rupture the labyrinthine window. This alone causes hearing loss, but more serious damage can be caused to the labyrinth if eardrops enter the cochlea at the same time.

(3) Before eardrops are administered, a test should be given to measure hearing in the high frequencies such as at 8,000 and 4,000 Hz. Tinnitus is often recognized by a patient; there are many patients, however, who do not feel tinnitus even at a considerably advanced stage of hearing loss.

(4) By using eardrops, a patient at times feels that his hearing has been improved temporarily. This is due to the fact that the round window membrane has been sealed by the drug solution, but the sensed improvement becomes the reason for the continuous use of the eardrops. This response,

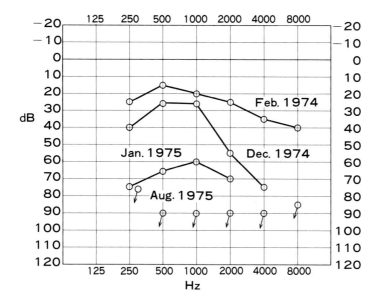

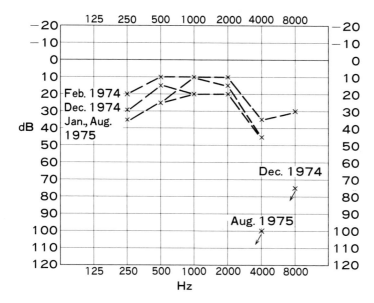

Fig. 61. Drug-induced hearing loss in a patient. Eardrops had been used for 7 months before they were stopped in December 1974. Hearing loss progressed even after the use of eardrops was stopped.

Table X. List of eardrops currently used in Japan

Trade name	Antibiotics	Anti-inflammatory agent	Stabilizer	Preservative	pH	Others
Chloromycetin (Sankyo Co., Ltd.)	chloramphenicol 5 mg (titer)					propylene glycol (dissolvent) ethyl aminobenzoate (analgesic and anti-pruritic actions)
Rinderon A (Shionogi Co., Ltd.)	fradiomycin sulfate 3.5 mg (titer)	betamethasone disodium phosphate 1 mg	dry sodium sulfite 2 mg	methyl para-oxybenzoate 0.5 mg	5.0–7.5	
Terra-Cortril Eye/Ear Suspension (Pfizer Taito Co., Ltd.)	oxytetracycline hydrochloride 5 mg (titer)	hydrocortisone acetate 15 mg				stearic acid (suspension) 20.2 mg liquid paraffin (lipophiric base) appropriate dose
Kanamycin (Meiji Seika Kaisha, Ltd.)	kanamycin sulfate 20 mg (titer)		sodium citrate 14 mg sodium bisulfite 5 mg	methyl para-oxybenzoate 0.9 mg propyl para-oxybenzoate 0.1 mg	4.8–5.0	
Orgadrone (Nippon Organon K.K.)		phosphoric dexamethasone-2-sodium 1 mg		benzalkonium chloride 0.1 mg	7.8–8.4	disodium edetate (anticoloring agent) boric acid, borax (buffer agent) sodium chloride (isotonic agent)

				pH	
Decadron (Nippon Merck Banyu Co., Ltd.)	dexamethasone sodium phosphate 1 mg	sodium bisulfite creatinine	benzalkonium chloride phenylethyl alcohol	7.2–7.8	disodium edetate (anticoloring agent) sodium citrate (isotonic agent) borax (buffer agent) polysorbate (surface-active agent) hydrochloric acid (pH adjusted)
Dexa-Scheroson (Nippon Schering Co., Ltd.)	dexamethasone sodium sulfate 1.26 mg (1 mg dexamethasone)		methyl paraoxybenzoate propyl paraoxybenzoate	6.3–7.2	
Chondron Dexa (Kaken Pharmaceutical Co., Ltd.)	dexamethasone sodium metasulfobenzoate		chlorobutanol 3.5 mg	5.0–7.0	sodium chondroitic acid (tissue activator)
Rinderon (Shionogi Co., Ltd.)	betamethasone disodium phosphate 1 mg	dry sodium sulfite 2 mg	methyl paraoxy-benzoate 0.5 mg propyl paraoxy-benzoate 0.2 mg	7.5–8.5	

Figures in this table show weights per milliliter.

however, provides the greatest risk of causing drug-induced hearing losses, because the drug solution is in continuous direct contact with the round window membrane.

(5) A continuous use of eardrops ought to be avoided. If no positive effect is seen after using eardrops for 7–10 days, their continuation will be useless.

Eardrops differ in purpose. Table X describes all eardrops currently used in Japan.

Lesions in the Cochlea Caused by the Use of Fradiomycin

An animal experiment was conducted to determine if fradiomycin would permeate the round window membrane and cause lesions in the cochlea. The experiment was made in two situations: when fradiomycin was placed directly on normal round window membranes, and when it was placed on round window membranes with experimentally induced serous otitis media.

Experiment 1: Round Window Membrane Permeability to Fradiomycin
Guinea pigs (200–300 g) with a normal Preyer's reflex were used for the experiment. Under nembutal anesthesia, the tympanic bulla was opened from the posterior portion of the ear to expose the round window membrane in a clear view. A small piece of gelfoam was dipped into physiological saline solution, having been made to absorb approximately 5 mg of powdered fradiomycin. This piece of gelfoam was placed directly onto the round window membrane. The opening in the posterior portion of the ear was temporarily closed by suturing.

As controls, ears treated with gelfoam dipped in only physiological saline solution were used. The guinea pigs were decapitated 1, 8 or 10 days after the operation. The tympanic bulla was taken out, fixed in 2.5% solution of glutaraldehyde, refixed in 1% solution of osmic acid and embedded in Epon. Samples were taken from each turn of the cochlea, from which sections with approximately 5 μm thickness were made. The sections were stained with toluidine blue, and were studied under a light microscope.

The cochleas of 10 ears were subjected to observation. Some of the samples taken from guinea pigs decapitated 1 day after the operation already showed degeneration of the hair cells. Those decapitated 8 days after the operation showed that the external hair cells had degenerated or disappeared, but the internal hair cells were intact. In those decapitated 10 days after the operation, the specimens revealed collapse of the spiral organ and disappearance of the internal and external hair cells.

Pathological changes in the spiral organ were most clearly observed in the basal turn and, in general, became less and less noticeable toward the upper turns. In addition, the external hair cells were more often damaged than the internal hair cells. Even when serious damage to the spiral organ was observed, the stria vascularis did not show any sign of pathological changes.

In general, the longer the interval between the operation and the decapitation, the more serious the pathological changes observed. There were some exceptions, however, showing considerable differences in the degree of pathological changes among all inner ears. On the other hand, there were no pathological changes detected in any of the control ear specimens.

Experiment 2: Influence of Lesions Pertaining to the Middle Ear

Guinea pigs (200–300 g) with a normal Preyer's reflex were used for the experiment. Under nembutal anesthesia, the soft palate of the guinea pig was incised to expose the pharyngeal orifice of the Eustachian tube under direct view. A small piece of silicone sponge was stuffed into the orifice to obstruct the Eustachian tube. In a separate group of guinea pigs, the tympanic bulla was opened from the inferior portion to obstruct the tympanic orifice of the Eustachian tube with epoxy resin. When the tympanic bulla was opened from the posterior portion of the ear 4–7 days after the operation, many ears had a pool of fluid inside the middle ear. Thus, serous otitis media was induced, and the experiment moved on to the next stage.

Using guinea pigs with serous otitis media of the left ear and a normal right ear (control ear), fradiomycin was placed on the round windows of both the left and right ears as described above. The day after the operation, the guinea pigs were decapitated; the tympanic bullae were removed and specimens were made from them.

In 9 guinea pigs, pathological changes of the cochlea were detected both in ears with serous otitis media and in control ears. In 7 guinea pigs, pathological changes of the cochlea were undetectable or detected only to a slight degree in ears with serous otitis media. All 7 animals, however, showed rather serious pathological changes in the cochleas of the control ears. In only 2 guinea pigs were pathological changes in the cochlea of the ear with serous otitis media more serious than those in the cochlea of the control ear.

Figure 62 shows the basal turn of the serous otitis media ear side of guinea pig No. 3, which did not show any pathological changes. Figure 63 is the control ear side of the same guinea pig, showing degeneration and disap-

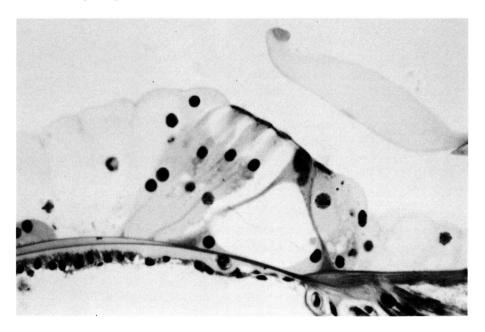

Fig. 62. The basal turn on the otitis media ear side. No pathological alteration is seen (guinea pig No. 3).

pearance of the internal and external hair cells. The basal turn on the serous otitis media ear side of guinea pig No. 8 shows its spiral organ completely destroyed due to serious pathological changes, but no abnormal changes in the stria vascularis were detected. Figure 64 is the second turn of the same cochlea. Pathological changes in the spiral organ are less serious than those in the basal turn, but the external hair cells were either degenerated or had disappeared. Figure 65 shows the same guinea pig's basal turn on the control ear side, which shows degeneration and disappearance of the external hair cells. This guinea pig showed more serious pathological changes of the cochlea in the ear with serous otitis media than in the control ear.

Thus, pathological changes of the cochlea were recognized after placing fradiomycin on the round window membrane. The pathological changes were localized in the spiral organ; more marked changes were seen in the basal turn than in the upper turns in general, and the external hair cells were more susceptible to damage than the internal hair cells.

Most ears with serous otitis media did not show any pathological changes in the cochlea; even when such changes occurred, they were very mild. On

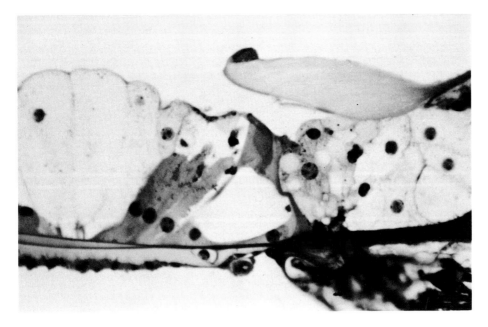

Fig. 63. The basal turn on the control ear side. Degeneration or disappearance is seen in the internal and external hair cells (guinea pig No. 3).

the other hand, all control ears showed pathological changes in the cochlea. 2 experimental animals showed more serious pathological changes in the cochlea on the serous otitis media ear side than in the cochlea on the control ear side. Findings of cochlear lesions were the same as those detected in experiment 1.

There are some reports on animal experiments in which fradiomycin was injected into the tympanic cavity. *Riskaer* et al. [1956] injected fradiomycin for as long as 30 days into the middle ear of guinea pigs with perforations experimentally produced in the tympanic membrane. Histological investigations were not conducted since there were no changes in the hearing of the guinea pigs. *Mittelman* [1972] did not detect any histological changes in the labyrinth in an experiment in which he introduced fradiomycin into the round window membrane once. *Kohonen and Tarkkanen* [1969] injected fradiomycin into the middle ears of guinea pigs, and classified the pathological changes in the labyrinth into three patterns. *Brummett* et al. [1976] also conducted the same experiment, and recognized the disappearance of the internal and external hair cells in all turns of the cochlea. *Nakai* et al. [1974]

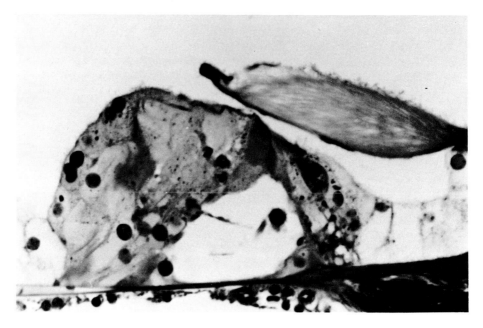

Fig. 64. The second turn on the otitis media ear side. Degeneration or disappearance is seen in the external hair cells. Pathological alteration is milder than in the basal turn (guinea pig No. 8).

injected eardrops containing fradiomycin and other ototoxic drugs into the tympanic cavities of monkeys and guinea pigs. They detected marked pathological changes in the external hair cells of the lower turns and in the internal hair cells and stria vascularis of the upper turns; they emphasized, at the same time, that there were great differences in pathological changes among animal species.

The results of experiment 1 indicate that pathological alteration in the cochlea is caused by placing fradiomycin directly on the round window membrane. This proves indirectly that round window membranes are permeable to fradiomycin, the same conclusion obtained in some of the aforementioned experiments. The present experiment showed that the pathological alteration induced by fradiomycin was more obvious in the basal turn than in the upper turns, and that the external hair cells were more susceptible to damage than the internal hair cells. It was observed in some experimental animals that in the apical turn the external hair cells survived, while the internal hair cells had disappeared; this finding was not omnipresent though. Such discrepan-

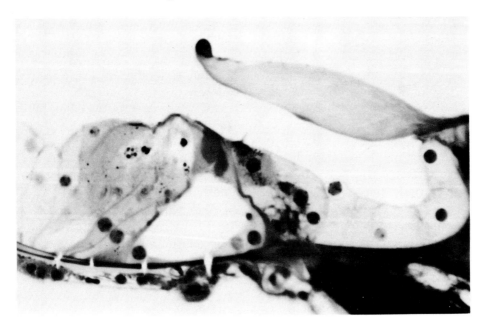

Fig. 65. The basal turn on the control ear side. Pathological alteration is less obvious than in the basal turn on the otitis media ear side (guinea pig No. 8).

cies in results obtained by different researchers are believed to be due to variations in experimental animals and conditions. Placing fradiomycin directly on the round window membrane, as in the present experiment, is unprecedented. With this method it is difficult to standardize the quantity of fradiomycin directly working on the round window membrane. However, it is possible that the drug works on the round window membrane for a relatively long period of time.

Incidentally, it is clinically well known that labyrinthitis often follows otitis media, and it has been found through histological investigations of the temporal bone that inflammation of the middle ear affects the round window membrane and diffuses directly into the labyrinth [*Paparella and Sugiura*, 1967]. Judging from observations of the oval window and the round window of animals with experimentally induced serous otitis media, *Goycoolea* et al. [1980c] predicted that round window membrane permeability increases in otitis media. *Goycoolea* et al. [1980b] demonstrated that round window permeability to albumin increases in experimentally induced serous otitis media.

They also recognized the passage of the exotoxin into the perilymph not only in ears with serous otitis media but also in normal ears, through an experiment using Staphylococcus exotoxin.

In contrast with these results, the result of the present experiment showed that pathological alteration of the labyrinth on the serous otitis media ear side was rarer. The following are the likely reasons for our experimental result: (1) Effusions prevent pools of fradiomycin on the round window membrane, thus reducing the permeation of fradiomycin from the middle ear to the inner ear. (2) Some chemical substances in the effusions combine with fradiomycin, thus neutralizing the ototoxic effects. (3) A defense mechanism is established within the tissue of the round window membrane.

There were, however, some clinical cases with serous otitis media in which severe sensorineural hearing loss occurred as a result of eardrop medication. Accordingly, further investigation is required concerning drug-induced hearing loss.

Round Window Membrane Rupture

At times the perilymph seeps out into the tympanic cavity. There are various factors causing this pathology. They occur in the oval window and/or the round window, and are called 'perilymphatic fistulae', 'labyrinthine window ruptures' and so on, taking into consideration the location and the causes of fistulae. The following names have been used in the literature: perilymphatic fistula (spontaneous, traumatic, vestibular); perilymph fistula; perilymphatic leaks; labyrinthine window ruptures; rupture of inner ear window; round window rupture; round window rupture syndrome; round window membrane rupture; round window fistula; rupture of the round window membrane.

Perilymphatic fistulae may be caused by various types of malformations, syphilis, otitis media, sequelae of otosclerosis surgery and a variety of traumas (including barotrauma). There are a significant number of cases where the causes are unknown: these are the so-called spontaneous perilymphatic fistulae.

In 1968, *Fee* conducted tympanotomy in cases with head trauma. He closely examined cases in which the oval window was disrupted, and emphasized in his report that perilymphatic fistulae were observed in nonoperated ears, thereby questioning the previous supposition that fistulae occur only following stapedectomy.

In 1971, *Goodhill* reported on a clinical case in which a perilymphatic fistula occurred, resulting in sudden hearing loss. He explained that fistulae were caused in the labyrinthine window via the explosive route created by an increase in cerebrospinal fluid pressure and the implosive route created by an increase in middle ear pressure.

Since *Fee's* [1968] report, a number of cases with labyrinthine window ruptures have been reported. During the 13-year period ending in 1981, at least 134 cases were reported in documents, of which 70 were oval window ruptures, 49 round window ruptures and 15 ruptures in both windows. It seems that the round window is less likely to rupture than the oval window.

A review of the reported cases of labyrinthine window rupture reveals that most ruptures occurred in those with a history of head trauma. These head traumas were caused not only by traffic accidents and other direct causes, but also by comparatively minor injuries such as falling or blows to the head. It is thus important to obtain sufficient information through questioning of the patient. The second largest number of ruptures occurred as a result of sudden changes of air pressure (barotrauma). These barometric changes were often caused by diving or flying; it should be noted, however, that many ruptures were also caused by sneezing, nose-blowing, carrying heavy objects, singing aloud or other actions considered rather ordinary in the course of everyday life. Labyrinthine window ruptures due to head trauma or barotrauma comprised approximately 70%, or slightly less, of all such ruptures. Although there were some cases where perilymphatic fistulae were caused by infection, the causes of about 30% of the ruptures are still unclear.

As one of the causes of labyrinthine window ruptures, anatomical properties have been mentioned; these include large cochlear aqueduct, absence of the round window niche, large round window and defective stapedial muscle.

Labyrinthine window ruptures have been shown to cause symptoms such as sensorineural hearing loss, tinnitus, vertigo and disequilibrium. Documents of patients that describe their history of illness in detail show that most cases of hearing loss are of the sudden type. In some cases, hearing fluctuates or further deteriorates to varying degrees; most cases do show, however, that hearing is impaired most frequently in the high frequencies.

Most patients suffering from tinnitus described the noise they heard with unique descriptions such as 'a streaming water-like sound'. Those noises are seemingly different from the continuous sound that is heard in cases of common sensorineural hearing loss.

Most vestibular symptoms appear first with paroxysmal rotatory vertigo. Close examination showed that there were many cases where positional nystagmus was experienced; dizziness, too, seemed to increase in certain head positions. Most cases of oval window fistulae reveal positive fistula signs while few cases of round window membrane fistulae do. Patients sometimes complain that they hear the sound of membrane breaking (a popping sound).

A diagnosis should be made keeping in mind the likelihood of labyrinthine window rupture. Round window membrane rupture is recognized less frequently than oval window rupture. Although there are differences in their respective clinical pictures, the possibility of such ruptures ought to be kept utmost in mind when encountering cases of sudden hearing loss, progressive sensorineural hearing loss of unknown causes, or fluctuating sensorineural hearing loss.

The first thing to be remembered in treating patients with labyrinthine window ruptures is to make sure they get strict bed rest. Resting with the head elevated at a 30° angle for 3–7 days can often cure these ruptures spontaneously. It should be noted that Valsalva's maneuver, Politzer's method and nose-blowing are to be avoided since such actions increase the cerebrospinal fluid pressure and the tympanic pressure.

When no sign of improvement is seen after 4 or 5 days' to a week's strict bed rest, surgery should be attempted. During a tympanotomy, the oval window and the round window are observed in order to detect perilymphatic leaks under a microscope. Perilymphatic leaks vary from case to case, described in documents as 'dripping out', 'slow seepage', 'seeping', 'welling up', 'oozing', 'streaming', 'free flowing' and so on. When the leak is not clear, it should be observed under a surgical microscope ($\times 25$, $\times 40$) for about 20 min. It has also been reported that the diagnosis should be made by using dry gelfoam, by making the patient use Valsalva's maneuver, by pressing the jugular vein, or by letting the patient take the Trendelenburg position. Tissue fluids that ooze out after removal of strands of connective tissues should be distinguished from perilymph. As for the round window membrane, singular or plural perforations, defective membrane, and linear slits have been described in patients with perilymphatic fistulae.

As mentioned in chapter 4, 70% of the temporal bones showed a membranous structure in the round window niche, and some of these were perforated. Taking into consideration that the actual round window membrane is hardly observable by tympanotomy, it is clear that the diagnosis ought to be made especially carefully.

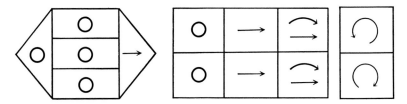

Fig. 66. Nystagmus before the operation.

Goodhill [1981] stated that round window membrane ruptures usually do not show as holes; rather they appear in the form of seepage in the inferior portion of the round window niche. As material for plugging the fistula, earlobe fat or fascia, connective tissue, vein graft or perichondrium graft, or gelfoam is used. Although gelfoam cures fistulae in a state close to the natural round window membrane, tissue grafts are considered better suited for divers. The bony margin of the round window niche is drilled, followed by the placing of a sealing material by lightly scratching the margin of the perforation. If the disrupted portion is not visible, the fistula can be sealed off by placing gelfoam only on its circumference.

Surgical intervention in the repair of labyrinthine window ruptures frequently provides an effective control of vertigo and disequilibrium. Hearing, however, cannot be improved much at times. Recurrences of labyrinthine window ruptures have been reported. The following case is an example of round window membrane rupture:

Subject T.T., a 16-year-old male high school student. This patient had been healthy since birth without any history of ear diseases. On September 5, 1979, however, he noticed a feeling of stuffiness and hearing loss in his right ear, both of which directly followed his standing on his head as he sang aloud in school. He does not recall hearing an ear-popping sound. Approximately half an hour later, he experienced dizziness. This was nonrotary, making him feel as though he were being pulled to his right. 1 h later, nausea and vomiting started, rendering him unable to sleep throughout the night. On the following day, the symptoms improved slightly. Figure 66 shows the observation of nystagmus on the 3rd day.

On September 14, when the patient was examined for the first time, his chief complaints were hearing loss, dizziness and unsteadiness. As he walked or changed his head position, the feeling of being pulled to his right persisted. His tympanic membrane was normal, with no observation suggesting a fluid pool inside his tympanic cavity. The result of the hearing test showed sensorineural hearing loss of approximately 65 dB in his right ear; the figures of hearing loss intensity scaled out at 4,000 and 8,000 Hz. In the Romberg test, the patient fell to the right. With gait testing, too, he leaned to his right after 4–5 steps, thereby making it impossible to continue the test.

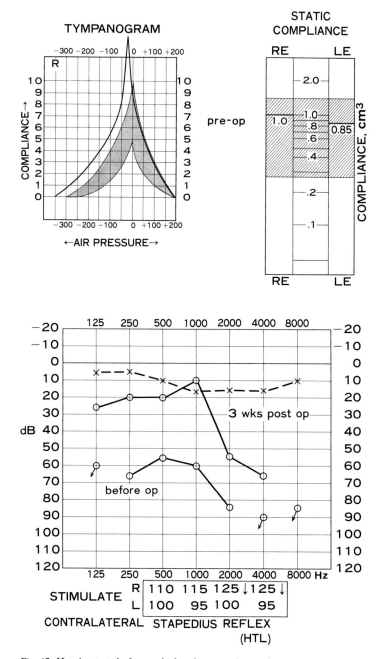

Fig. 67.: Hearing tests before and after the operation.

On September 17, 12 days after the onset of the symptoms, an exploratory tympanotomy was conducted on his right ear. While no changes were detected in the circumference of the stapes, under the microscope, fluid was observed running from the round window niche to the hypotympanum proper, the flow increasing as the jugular vein was compressed. Although the round window membrane could be partially seen, the fistula remained invisible. Without drilling the bony margin of the round window niche, the mucoperiosteum was partially scratched. After insertion of gelfoam, the elevated tympanic membrane was returned to the original position to complete the surgery. For 3 days after the surgery, the patient was kept in the reclining position at 30°.

At the time the patient left the hospital on October 1, neither spontaneous nystagmus nor positional nystagmus was observed. Dizziness had been alleviated significantly. Figure 67 shows the audiograms taken before and after surgery.

Experimentally Induced Round Window Membrane Rupture

Using temporal bones of humans and guinea pigs, an experiment was conducted with regard to round window membrane rupture. The objective of this experiment was to determine the pressure required to cause round window membrane rupture, the state/shape of the ruptured sites, and so on.

Humans

Applying Pressure through the Cochlear Aqueduct

Adult temporal bones from 25 ears were used. A thin needle (outer diameter 0.61 mm, inner diameter 0.47 mm) was inserted from the external aperture of the cochlear aqueduct. An injector that contained diluted Recorder Ink (Right Co., Ltd.) was connected to the needle, and pressure was applied by strongly forcing it towards the running direction of the cochlear aqueduct. This procedure was conducted under a surgical microscope in order to observe any ink seepage from either the oval window or the round window. The results are shown in table XI. In temporal bones in which fistulae did not occur, more than 300 mm Hg of pressure was applied on their cochlear aqueducts. In those in which fistulae occurred either in the oval window or the round window, fistulae were caused at less pressure. Once fistulae were formed, furthermore, dye solution seeped out without resistance. The rupture sites and their shapes will be discussed later.

Table XI. Injection of dye solution through the cochlear aqueduct (25 ears)

	Ears, n
Temporal bones with dye inside the cochlea	12
Oval window ruptures	3
Round window ruptures	2
No ruptures	7
Temporal bones without dye inside the cochlea	13

Table XII. Injection of dye solution to the scala tympani (10 ears)

	Ears, n
Oval window ruptures	7
Round window membrane ruptures	2
No ruptures	1

Applying Pressure through the Scala Tympani

Temporal bones from 10 ears were used. A small hole was punctured in the scala tympani at the basal turn near the round window membrane using a bur of 0.5 mm diameter. A two-step needle (outer diameter of the tip 0.37 mm, inner diameter 0.18 mm, length 2 mm) was inserted into the hole and was secured with dental cement (G-C Dental Industrial Corp.). Pressure was applied to the cochlea in the same method as previously described in order to see whether the membranes would rupture or not. The results are shown in table XII.

Of oval window ruptures, three were found to have occurred in the superomedial portion of the annular ligament, three in the inferomedial portion and the remaining one in the posterior portion.

Fig. 68. a, b. Human round window membrane rupture. Although the slit runs in the direction of the fibers, the fibers do not simply run in the same direction. *b* is a high-power view of *a*.

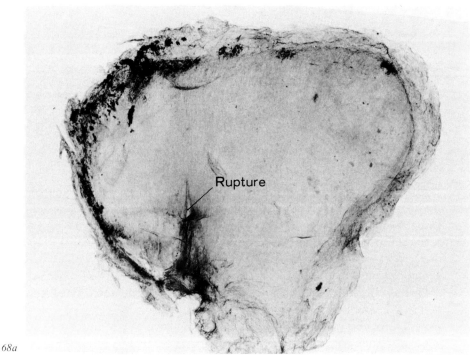

Rupture

68a

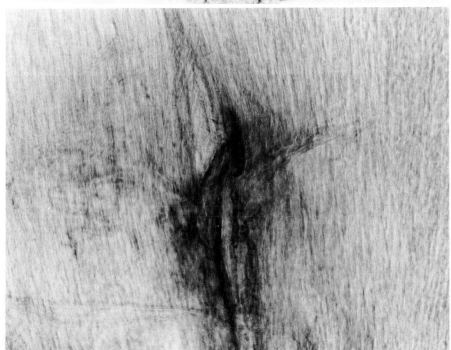

68b

Round window membrane ruptures were seen in ears having had pressure applied, two through the cochlear aqueduct and two through the scala tympani. All four ears showed slit-like fistulae running parallel to the direction of the round window membrane fibers. Round fistulae were not detected (fig. 68a, b).

Guinea Pigs
Applying Pressure through the Scala Tympani

14 albino guinea pigs weighing 200–300 g were used. All these animals showed a normal Preyer's reflex and were not suffering from otitis media. Under nembutal anesthesia, a small hole was punctured in the scala tympani of the left cochlear basal turn using a bur. A glass capillary tube with 0.7 mm diameter at the tip was inserted into the scala tympani and was secured with dental cement. The tube was connected to a three-way cock. The other site of the cock was attached to an inner ear pressure manometer (Natsume Mfg.) utilizing a semiconductor membrane pressure sensor, as well as an X-Y recorder, for recording (fig. 69). The remaining cock was connected to an injector containing artificial perilymph (10 mM NaHCO$_3$, 130 mM NaCl, 4 mM KCl, 1.5 mM CaCl$_2$, 1 mM MgCl$_2$, 20 mM Hepes-HCl pH 7.4, 150 mM phosphate buffer solution pH 7.4) to apply pressure. It was positioned so that this liquid would enter the cochlea.

Results

Approximately 100 mm H$_2$O of pressure was recorded when the manometer was connected to the cochlea. When pressure gradients were increased by 200 mm H$_2$O/min, 10 of the 14 ears showed leakage from the labyrinthine window. 3 of the 10 ears exhibited a welling up of fluid at the joint between the capillary tube and the cochlea, while the tip of the capillary tube attached to one ear had been closed off.

Of the 10 ears that showed labyrinthine window ruptures, 9 showed round window membrane ruptures and the other one showed an oval window rupture. 8 of the 9 ears had oblong ruptures in the inferior margin of the round window membrane, running in the direction of the fibers. One ear showed a slit-like rupture. Pressures at which ruptures were caused were over 400 mm H$_2$O for 9 out of 10 ears, while the other one showed round window membrane rupture at 220 mm H$_2$O. There were ears which did not rupture even at 1,200 mm H$_2$O.

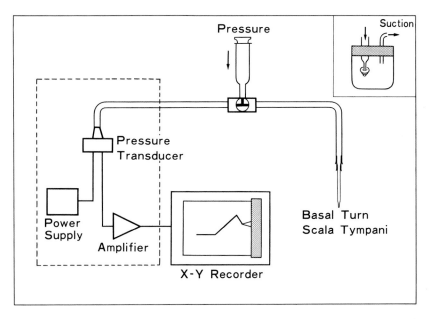

Fig. 69. Measuring the labyrinthine pressure. In the insert of the diagram, a beaker takes the place of the middle ear. A removed cochlea is placed in the beaker. The experiment is conducted by adding pressure to the scala tympani and by lowering the pressure in the beaker (negative pressure).

Effects of Negative Tympanic Pressure on Labyrinthine Window Ruptures

When pressure is applied to the cochlea, the pressure gradient becomes higher in the labyrinthine window if the inside of the tympanic cavity shows negative pressure. The following experiment was conducted, using removed temporal bones. A 20-ml glass beaker was covered and sealed air-tight. The beaker was furnished with a tube to adjust the pressure inside the beaker, as well as a glass capillary tube to be inserted into the cochlea, as in the previously described experiment (fig. 69, insert).

The cochlear aqueduct and the internal auditory meatus of the temporal bone were sealed off with cement, while a glass capillary tube was inserted into a small hole pierced through the scala tympani at the basal turn. The glass capillary tube was secured with dental cement and connected to an inner ear pressure manometer and to an X-Y recorder (fig. 69).

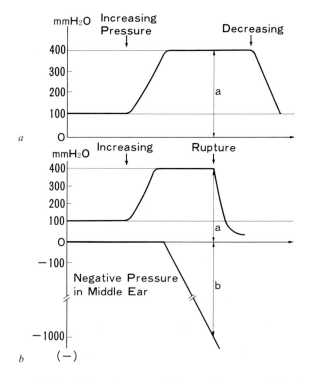

Fig. 70.a, b. Experiment combining positive pressure in the inner ear and negative pressure in the middle ear. *a* No ruptures were detected, despite 400 mm H_2O of pressure on the round window membrane. *b* Over 1,000 mm H_2O of negative pressure on the tympanic cavity, giving a total of over 1,400 mm H_2O of pressure (a + b) on the round window membrane. As a result, the round window membrane ruptured.

The cochlea was subjected to increasing pressure gradients up to a maximum of 400 mm H_2O in 3 guinea pigs, but no rupture was noted. Adjusting the beaker pressure to − 300 mm H_2O did not cause any ruptures either, nor did readjusting the same pressure suddenly to 0. However, when 400 mm H_2O of pressure was applied to the cochlea, in addition to more than − 1,000 mm H_2O of negative pressure applied to the beaker, the round window membrane showed ruptures (fig. 70a, b).

In reference to labyrinthine window ruptures, what *Goodhill* [1971] referred to as 'the explosive route' is the theory that an increase in cerebrospinal fluid pressure would influence the inner ear to cause ruptures. Several factors, such as the degree of the cochlear aqueduct's patency, pressure through the internal auditory meatus, hydrodynamic force of labyrinthine venous fluid, and so on, are also responsible for such membrane ruptures.

The present experiment was conducted using human temporal bones to see whether the round window membrane would rupture on the application of pressure through the cochlear aqueduct. This experiment was designed to investigate the explosive route.

Reports on the patency of the human cochlear aqueduct do not necessarily agree with one another. For instance, *Palva and Dammert* [1969] stated that it was patent, while *Ritter and Lawrence* [1965] insisted that the human cochlear aqueduct was narrow and filled with connective tissue, allowing no free communication between the cerebrospinal fluid and the perilymph. These authors reported, furthermore, that radioiodinated serum albumin and a dye stuff (indigo carmine) injected intrathecally could not be detected in the perilymph in clinical cases. *Holden and Schuknecht* [1968] noted wide cochlear aqueducts in 6 out of 12 temporal bones with subarachnoidal hemorrhage. Erythrocytes had passed into the cochlea through the wide cochlear aqueduct. *Rask-Andersen* et al. [1977] noted that 79 out of 82 temporal bones examined had patent cochlear aqueducts, while the remaining three temporal bones had sealed cochlear aqueducts with the jugular fossa located in significantly high positions.

In the present experiment, a dye solution was injected via the cochlear aqueduct. Of the 25 temporal bones observed, 12 (48%) showed the presence of dye but 13 did not. Although there might have been some technical problems, the fact that several attempts were made with substantial pressure each time suggests that those temporal bones not allowing the passage of the dye solution show poor patency of the cochlear aqueduct. There were no temporal bones which showed dye solution seepage via the internal auditory meatus.

The width of the cochlear aqueduct varies between adults and children: an adult's diameter of 100 μm contrasts with a child's 150 μm [*Palva*, 1970]. It can therefore be said that via the explosive route, it is easy to apply pressure through the infant's cochlear aqueduct to the inner ear. There are many reports of labyrinthine window ruptures in children. In examining a child reporting hearing loss, dizziness or disequilibrium, the possibility of labyrinthine window ruptures cannot be overlooked.

There is an old report by *Meurman* [1929] on the relationship between cerebrospinal pressure and inner ear pressure based on animal experiments. He confirmed that by increasing the cerebrospinal pressure in rabbits, the pressure of the scala tympani, too, was increased. Recent experiments also showed that inner ear pressure is almost equal to cerebrospinal pressure, and that changes in cerebrospinal pressure affect the inner ear [*Kerth and Allen*, 1963; *Beentjes*, 1972; *Myers*, 1973].

In experiments, pressures at which labyrinthine window ruptures were caused varied considerably. For example, although *Miriszlai and Sándor* [1980] noted ruptures at 23.4 mm Hg on average in cats, there were some cats in which ruptures did not occur at 230 mm Hg, and yet others whose labyrinthine window ruptured at 6 mm Hg.

In the present experiment using guinea pigs, most of the animals required over 400 mm H_2O for their windows to rupture, but there were also some animals in which ruptures occurred at 220 mm H_2O. Pressure was applied via the scala tympani in all the guinea pigs, but the width of the cochlear aqueduct, the pressure velocity, and the vulnerability of the membrane itself are all relevant factors. It is believed that the number of fibers in the middle layer of the round window membrane and their order influence ruptures. Ruptures, as seen in guinea pigs, often occur along the running direction of fibers, just as in humans.

Study of previous reports on animal experiments shows that round window ruptures were noted in almost all experiments. However, there is no description of oval window rupture [*Harker* et al. 1974; *Miriszlai and Sándor*, 1980]. In our experiment, oval window rupture was noted in 1 of the 10 guinea pigs. In the experiment using human temporal bones, pressures were applied either via the cochlear aqueduct or via the scala tympani, and the oval window/round window ratios were 3:2/7:2, respectively, in terms of the location and the frequency of ruptures. These figures support the fact that oval window rupture is encountered clinically more frequently than round window rupture.

It is not rare for the tympanic cavity to have negative pressure. According to *Magnuson* [1981], negative pressure on the middle ear caused by sniffing as normal people do was − 140 mm H_2O on average and − 400 mm H_2O at maximum. He further stated that subjects with poor Eustachian tube functions showed negative pressure up to − 1,200 mm H_2O in the same situation. As the tympanic pressure becomes negative, the round window membrane should have the same amount of pressure added in excess of the cerebrospinal fluid pressure. The present experiment also showed that when the tympanic pressure turned negative, round window ruptures occurred even at inner ear pressures not normally high enough to cause ruptures.

What would happen if the round window membrane ruptured in cases of serous otitis media? How would hearing be influenced? These issues will be dealt with in the next section.

Experimental Round Window Membrane Rupture

A Time-Course Observation of Cochlear Potential in Both Normal Ears and Ears with Serous Otitis Media after Round Window Membrane Ruptures

Labyrinthine window ruptures and the formation of perilymphatic fistulae as a result of such ruptures are considered to be one of the causes of sudden hearing loss. It is doubtful, however, that a simple perilymphatic fistula causes sensorineural hearing loss. For the purpose of examining this point, round window membranes were incised in normal ears to make a time-course observation of their cochlear potentials.

Clinically progressive sensorineural hearing loss occurs in patients with serous otitis media without apparent cause. Although there are few reports on these cases and the mechanism of the pathogenesis has not been clarified, it can be considered that the occurrence of round window membrane rupture in cases with serous otitis media is a cause of the development of sensorineural hearing loss. To pursue this supposition, round window membranes were experimentally incised in ears with experimentally induced serous otitis media to make time-course observations of cochlear potentials, just as the normal ears were examined.

Albino guinea pigs weighing 200–300 g, with a normal Preyer's reflex, were used in the present experiment. The guinea pigs were anesthetized with an intraperitoneal injection of pentobarbital at a dose of 40 mg/kg. In normal ear experiments, the round window membrane was exposed through the dorsolateral approach and was incised to about half of its diameter using a No. 27 gauge hypodermic needle tip. Perilymphatic leaks were found immediately after the incision. No material was placed on the membrane, and the skin was sutured.

To produce serous otitis media, the tympanic bulla was opened through the ventral side, and the Eustachian tube orifice was cauterized by applying 10% silver nitrate solution. Accumulation of serous sterile middle ear fluid was observed on the first day, and fluid was detected after 1 month as well. 5 days after the operation, the tympanic bulla was exposed through the dorsolateral approach and the round window membrane was incised in the same way as for the normal ears. In the process of this operation, the fluid in the middle ear space was sucked off. After the incision, the skin incision was sutured without any treatment on the membrane.

Throughout the postoperative course, cephalosporin (150 mg/kg) was administered. A silver wire (170 μm in diameter), coated with teflon except at the tip, was used as the different electrode. The tip of this wire was made into a ball 500 μm in diameter, and was fastened at the margin of the round window membrane. It was further secured to the tympanic bulla with dental cement above the silver ball. As indifferent and ground electrodes, silver-coated screws 500 μm in diameter were used; the indifferent electrode was placed in the frontal bone, the ground electrode in the occipital bone. A silver screw electrode was placed in the vertex to record the auditory-evoked brainstem responses (ABR).

Sound stimulus was presented via a 6.4-mm condenser microphone. The microphone was coupled tightly to the bony meatus. Short tone bursts and clicks were derived from an oscillator (DA-505, Dana Japan), and were amplified through an attenuator and an amplifier (SU-A8, Technics). Short tone bursts and clicks were calibrated in a 0.4-ml coupler. The evoked responses were connected to a differential amplifier (7S-11A, Sanei) ($\times 10^4$, band-pass: DC-3,000 Hz for AP, CM recordings, 160–3,000 Hz for ABR recordings) and were averaged.

In chronic experiments, granulations usually occur at the tip of the electrodes, inducing electric leaks and thereby deteriorating cochlear potentials. Therefore, 5 control (untreated) guinea pigs were used to follow the time-course changes, and the average of these values was used to correct the experimental data.

Electrophysiological measurements were carried out four times at 10-day intervals, before the membrane rupture and 10, 20 and 30 days after the rupture. On the 30th day, the experimental animals were decapitated and their temporal bones removed. The round window membranes, whether normal or with serous otitis media, were closed off completely in all the animals. Ten normal ears and six with serous otitis media were studied.

Normal Ears

The average values of the input/output curve of AP are shown in figure 71. Clicks were derived from 100-μs rectangular pulses. On the 10th day after the operation, elevation of the AP threshold level by approximately 20 dB and prolongation of the latency by 0.1–0.15 ms were demonstrated. The input/output curve obtained at 10 days after the operation was parallel to the

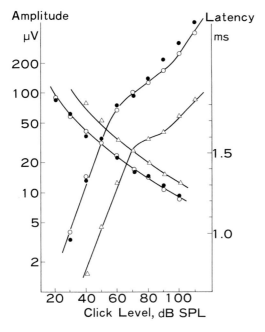

Fig. 71. Input/output curve of the AP. ○ = Before the operation; △ = 10 days after operation; ● = 30 days after operation. At 10 days after the operation, amplitude and latency of the AP revealed that conductive hearing loss had occurred. At 30 days after the operation, the levels returned to normal.

preoperative one. No signs of recruitment phenomena such as steep curves were detected. The AP waves taken at 10 days after the operation also showed the same shape as the preoperative ones. All these findings suggested that the changes detected 10 days following the operation showed conductive hearing loss. At 30 days after the operation, both the N1 amplitude and latency returned to approximately the same figures as before the operation.

In order to learn the frequency character in round window membrane ruptures, a study was made of changes in CM. Figure 72 shows the time-course changes in the frequency characteristics of CM. At 10 days after the operation, the threshold level was elevated by approximately 20 dB; particularly notable was the elevation in the high frequencies (fig. 72, arrow). At 30 days after the operation, any difference from before the operation was rarely detectable.

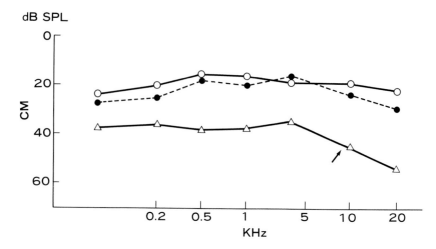

Fig. 72. CM detection levels. 10 days after the operation, there was a hearing loss of 10–20 dB on the average. This hearing loss was particularly noticeable at high frequencies (see arrow). Symbols are the same as those used in figure 71.

Ears with Serous Otitis Media

The ABR thresholds measured at 5 days after the Eustachian tube obstruction were 25 dB at 1,000 and 2,000 Hz, 30 dB at 4,000 Hz and 36 dB at 8,000 Hz. The input/output curves of AP at this time were consistent with conductive hearing loss. At 10 days after the round window membrane rupture, the ABR threshold level elevated by approximately 10 dB at 1,000 and 2,000 Hz, and over 20 dB at 4,000 and 8,000 Hz (fig. 73). At this time, the input/output curves of AP at the tone burst of 4,000 Hz showed only a steep H-curve and were positive, suggesting recruitment phenomenon. On the 30th day, the ABR threshold levels at low frequencies varied greatly from those at high frequencies. At 1,000 and 2,000 Hz, the ABR threshold level had been elevated by 5 dB from before the operation; at 4,000 and 8,000 Hz, however, the threshold level remained 10–15 dB worse than before the operation. The AP input/output curves at the 4,000 Hz tone burst 30 days after the operation were consistent with sensorineural hearing loss.

The incised round window membranes of both normal ears and those with serous otitis media were occluded completely by the 30th day after the operation. The incision of the round window membranes in normal ears caused temporary conductive hearing loss. As fluid was absorbed and the

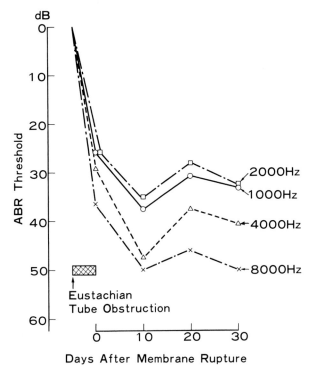

Fig. 73. Round window membrane ruptures in ears with experimental serous otitis media. No recovery of hearing was observed at 4,000 and 8,000 Hz, even 30 days after the operation.

round window membranes were sealed, hearing returned completely to normal. Severe hearing losses were, however, recognized in the high frequencies soon after the operation.

The present experiment shows that hearing loss due to round window rupture is temporary and hearing may return to normal. Clinically speaking, however, the prognosis for hearing in patients with round window rupture is not always good. This leads to the theory that round window membrane rupture is only a small part of the pathological changes, hiding more serious lesions inside the cochlea. In this regard, the name round window rupture syndrome [*Weisskopf* et al., 1978] is also used. The rupture of the membranous labyrinth and the various pathological changes resulting from it, as well as the healing process, must act as influential factors.

In the ears with serous otitis media, the ABR responses were depressed in all frequency regions after the rupture of the round window membrane. The input/output curve of the AP showed only an H-curve, and was compatible with sensorineural hearing loss. Although hearing showed an improvement at low frequencies 20 and 30 days after the operation, eventually returning to the same level as before the operation, the higher the frequency was, the less improvement the threshold levels showed. As a result, the sensorineural hearing loss was not completely reversed.

Round window membrane rupture could also occur in patients with serous otitis media. The tympanic pressure is not always negative in ears with serous otitis media. However, when the middle ear has a high negative pressure, a pressure gradient across the round window membrane becomes extremely high. Middle ear effusion has to be treated as soon as possible, otherwise patients run the risk of developing round window rupture.

Viral Labyrinthitis

Viruses could reach the inner ear via the hematogenous route or cerebrospinal fluid route. The former causes endolymphatic labyrinthitis, mainly causing pathological changes in the stria vascularis, while the latter causes perilymphatic (meningogenic) labyrinthitis. It is not known whether viruses cause labyrinthitis by entering the cochlea through the round window membrane. Experimentally induced viral labyrinthitis has been studied in detail by the Idiopathic Sensorineural Hearing Loss Research Group of the Intractable Diseases Division, Public Health Bureau, Ministry of Health and Welfare, Japan (led by Prof. *Hiroshi Miyake* of Nagoya University). It was reported by this group that pathological changes in the inner ear were caused by experimentally inoculated herpes simplex virus (HSV) and Sendai virus [*Terayama* et al., 1980; *Kurata* et al., 1982; *Koide* et al., 1982].

In the above experiments, viruses were injected directly into the cochlea. But when experiments were conducted using HSV to find whether viruses passed through the normal round window membrane into the inner ear, only negative results were obtained. An experiment was conducted using female

Fig. 74. Viral labyrinthitis (guinea pig). *a* There were no changes in the inner ear when virus was placed on the round window membrane. *b* After the virus was injected through the round window membrane into the scala tympani, viral labyrinthitis was detected.

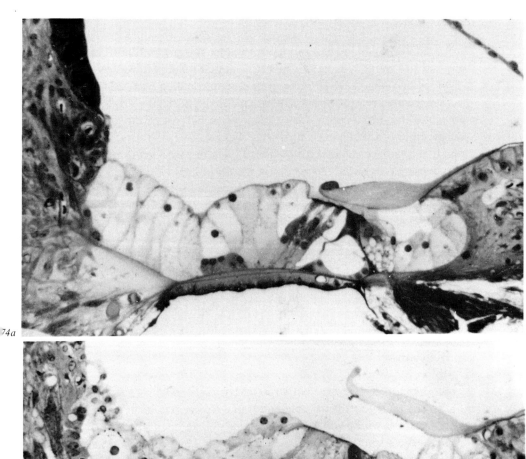

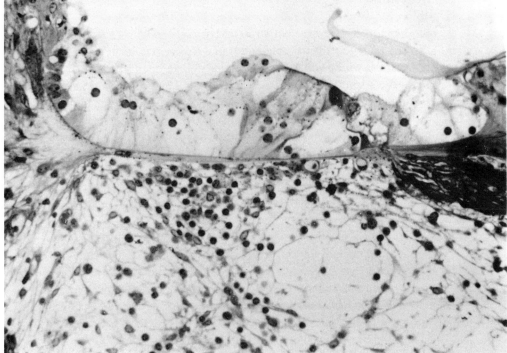

Hartley guinea pigs. Under nembutal anesthesia, the posterior portion of the right external auditory meatus was incised, and a small hole was pierced in the tympanic bulla. A small amount of gelfoam soaked with HSV 2×10^3 plaque-forming units (pfu)/0.002 ml was placed on the round window membrane, and the skin incision was sutured. After 6–18 days, the guinea pigs were decapitated to prepare samples. The virus was the HSV 2-type Ogiwara strain that had been isolated from a human neonate infected throughout its body, and a passage was carried out in the fibroblasts of a human embryo. The virus value was 1×10^6 pfu/ml in the undiluted solution.

Virus antigen was tested for by the indirect fluorescent antibody method; it was not detected in any of the animals. Figure 74a, b shows the specimens observed under a light microscope when the virus was placed on the round window membrane and when virus was injected directly into the scala tympani.

Otosclerosis and Anomaly

Otosclerosis

The vicinity of the round window is the area second most susceptible to otosclerosis, after the fissula antefenestram. A case has been reported in which the round window niche was occluded and an open surgery was conducted on the round window [*House and Glorig,* 1960]. Otosclerosis is categorized into two groups according to hearing loss: type I showing moderate hearing loss in all frequency regions, and type II showing a higher degree of hearing loss, especially progressive towards the high-frequency regions. Of 153 cases of round window otosclerosis, 107 were of type I and 46 were of type II [*Huygen* et al., 1974].

Anomaly

Anomaly of the labyrinthine window is considered to be extremely rare. Of all reports on histopathological studies of temporal bones, none focus on anomaly of the round window. Statistics taken from various documents on anomaly of the oval window show that about one-third of cases with congenitally defective oval windows also had round window defects [*Harada* et al., 1980]. It was, however, reported that some cases of labyrinthine anomaly showed normal stapes and that other cases had a complication of middle ear anomaly and oval window defect. In all the cases, hearing was improved by opening up the round window [*Harrison* et al., 1964; *Ombredanne*, 1968; *Richards*, 1981].

9. Via the Round Window Therapeutics for Ear Diseases

As already described, the round window is the route which connects the inner ear to the middle ear, and through which drugs diffuse into the inner ear. Accordingly, the round window can be useful when treating ear diseases. This pathway between the two compartments (middle and inner ear), however, has so far been involved more frequently in treating vertigo – in particular, Ménière's disease – than in treating hearing losses. In the future this pathway will be utilized in the treatment of hearing losses too. Shunt operations are included among the surgical methods which have been advocated for patients with Ménière's disease. In one type of shunt operation, the endolymph is made to communicate with the perilymph in order to reduce pressure.

Neurectomy of the posterior ampullary nerve is a surgical therapy for benign paroxysmal positional vertigo. This operation requires the dissection of the round window niche, since the singular nerve in this ampulla runs immediately beneath the round window membrane. In this chapter, therapeutic methods for ear diseases pertaining to the round window membrane and the round window niche will be discussed.

Ablation Therapy

The pathology of Ménière's disease is endolymphatic hydrops. Therapeutics for this disease vary from administering drugs to surgery for reducing pressure in the endolymph. A labyrinthectomy can be performed if hearing has seriously deteriorated. There are various methods for conducting labyrinthectomies. *Cawthorne* [1943] reported a method destroying the lateral semicircular canal, while *Lempert* [1948] described a decompression operation in which the round window membrane is broken after removing the stapes via the tympanic cavity. *Schuknecht* [1957] reported another method in which a part of the inner ear is removed after the oval window and the round window are opened. Although it is common to perform a labyrinthectomy by approaching the labyrinth from both windows, the surest procedure was reported by *Schuknecht and Hammerschlag* [1977]: the oval window is approached via the external auditory meatus, and the utricle is removed under the direct view. The three semicircular ampullae are destroyed through the oval window.

Schuknecht [1957] reported that the labyrinth would be destroyed by injecting streptomycin into the tympanic cavity. This therapy was developed based upon the facts that the vestibule is easily damaged by streptomycin sulfate and that little postmortem change is observed when 10% formalin is injected into the tympanic cavity at autopsy. In this therapy, a small incision is made in the inferior wall of the external auditory meatus, 3 mm lateral to the tympanic ring; then a tube is inserted from this incision, between the bony portion of the external auditory meatus and the tympanic ring, into the tympanic cavity so that the drug solution can be injected into the tympanic cavity without dissecting the tympanic membrane. The hair cells are damaged by this method when the streptomycin is diffused via the round window into the inner ear. If a drug is used which selectively damages the vestibular system, keeping the hair cells in the organ of Corti intact, the therapeutic purpose can be attained without causing hearing loss.

It is not certain that when a drug is injected into the inner ear to carry out destruction of the labyrinth, it also enters the opposite inner ear. *Schreiner* [1966] reported that ^{32}P injected into one side of the inner ear of animals rapidly diffused into the inner ear on the other side. It is unclear whether the drug solution passed through the cochlear aqueduct or through the perineural tissues. It is necessary to keep in mind that injected drug solutions may diffuse into the opposite inner ear during actual treatment.

Ultrasonic irradiation is included in a number of operations for treating Ménière's disease. In this method, an irradiation is performed from the round window towards the vestibulum and semicircular canals. Although the semicircular canal technique, in which the lateral semicircular canal was irradiated, was used at one time, this method required drilling into the mastoid antrum, risking hearing disturbance or facial paralysis. The round window technique, in which irradiation is performed via the round window, requires only one-tenth as much energy as the semicircular canal technique, resulting in fewer complications. It is possible to irradiate, via the round window, the saccule, the utricle, and the anterior and lateral semicircular canals and destroy them; at the same time, the cochlea can be kept intact, thanks to the anatomical relationship [*Kossoff* et al., 1967]. Many feel that ultrasonic irradiation via the round window is worth the attempt because it is less invasive than other surgical methods [*Pappas* et al., 1980].

Osmotic Induction Therapy

The osmotic induction method is a treatment method suggested by *Arslan* [1969, 1970, 1972], taking advantage of the semipermeability of the round window membrane. In this treatment, a desiccated, sterilized salt crystal of less than 1 mm in diameter is placed in the round window niche by elevating the tympanic membrane. The purpose of this treatment is to cure endolymphatic hydrops.

The direction of nystagmus changes as time passes. There is an irritative phase starting immediately after the operation, in which the nystagmus is directed towards the involved ear; later, the direction of nystagmus becomes reversed and beats towards the uninvolved, or healthy, ear. This later phase is called the paralytic phase. According to *Arslan*, in the irritative phase, a difference in osmotic pressure can be induced across the inside and outside of the round window membrane by placing a salt crystal in the round window niche, causing the cochlear duct to collapse as a result of water shifting to the middle ear from both the perilymph and the endolymph. During the paralytic phase, this loss of water from the perilymph is compensated rapidly through ultrafiltration, and a difference in osmotic pressure occurs between the perilymph and the endolymph. Since water is shifted from the perilymph to the endolymph, which is hyperosmotic, its volume is increased.

According to an analysis of the inner ear fluids, the irritative phase occurs because the receptors of the vestibule become excited as the K^+ level in the perilymph increases. The paralytic phase, on the other hand, is the result of compensational inhibition of the central system as the ionic composition returns to the normal state [*Molinari*, 1972].

In order to observe the changes in the inner ear, osmotic induction was attempted on rabbits. Under local anesthesia, the tympanic bulla was opened up and a salt crystal (approx. 0.5 g) was placed in the round window niche and covered with gelfoam; the opening was then sutured temporarily. For about 60 min after the operation, active nystagmus was observed towards the operated side (irritative phase); it then shifted direction to the nonoperated side. The nystagmus was most active 90 min after the operation (paralytic phase). These types of nystagmus were influenced by furosemide; the irrit-

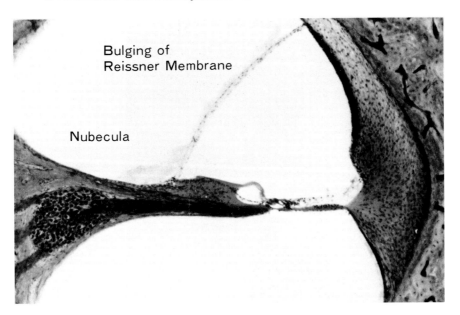

Bulging of
Reissner Membrane

Nubecula

Fig. 75. Cochlear changes through the osmotic induction method. A slight bulging of the Reissner's membrane is seen in the lower basal turn – irritative phase (rabbit).

ative phase, therefore, was suppressed, while the paralytic phase was prolonged [*Futaki* et al., 1980].

The inner ears were removed and fixed in order to prepare specimens during the irritative phase. A slight degree of bulging was detected in the Reissner's membrane at the lower basal turn; however, there was no sign of collapse (fig. 75). In any case, it is clear that the endocochlear potential becomes lower when salt is placed on the round window membrane, influencing stria vascularis [*Asakuma* et al., 1973]. Incidentally, *Fowler and Forbes* [1936] conducted an animal experiment using sodium chloride crystals and observed some changes in the spiral organ. They reported that hearing deteriorated when this method was used.

Cochlear Endolymphatic Shunt (Cochleosacculotomy)

Among a number of operations for treating Ménière's disease, there is one in which communication is opened between the endolymph and the perilymph; this endolymph-perilymph shunt operation aims at leakage of

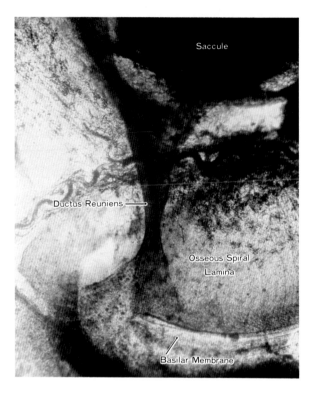

Fig. 76. Relationship between the terminal portion of the cochlea, ductus reuniens and saccule.

the excess endolymph fluid into the perilymph by creating a fistula in the endolymphatic system. Although several surgical methods have been advocated [*Fick*, 1964, 1966; *Cody* et al., 1967; *Cody*, 1969], none of them have obtained satisfactory results.

Pulec [1968] devised an otic-perotic shunt method. In this method, a platinum shunt tube (outer diameter 0.5 mm, inner diameter 0.35 mm, length 1 mm) is inserted into the basilar membrane via the round window membrane, aiming at connection of the scala media and the scala tympani. This method was found to have resulted in severe hearing loss in 25% of all cases. It has not been put into practice as a result [*Pulec*, 1969].

Based on a similar notion, *Schuknecht* [1981] conducted an operation in which he inserted a pick from the round window through the cochlea into the vestibule. The purpose of the operation was to create an eternal

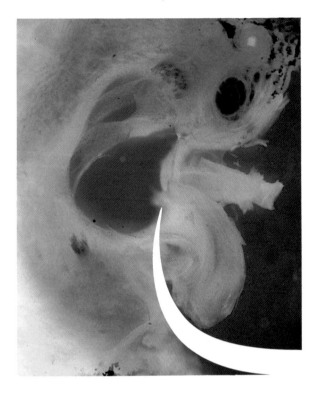

Fig. 77. Cochlear endolymphatic shunt. A pick (white area) is inserted through the round window membrane into the vestibule.

endolymphatic fistula, based on the results of animal experiments. In the case of Ménière's disease, if the saccule has a bulge, a fistula is created in the sac- cule by this operation, and its name, cochleosacculotomy, originated from this. However, this surgical procedure has come to be called cochlear endolymphatic shunt. If the saccule does not show any bulges, it is main- tained as it is; there is, however, a significant possibility that the ductus reuniens might be destroyed (fig. 76).

As a surgical method, a tympanomeatal flap is created under an oto- scope, and is elevated in order to open up the tympanic cavity. The bony rim of the round window is partly drilled to expose the round window membrane. A perpendicular or curved pick is inserted through the round window mem- brane 3 mm in the direction of the vestibule, or upward (fig. 77). After this operation, gelfoam is placed in the round window niche, followed by the replacement of the elevated tympanic membrane in its original position. This is a simple procedure because the affected site is limited to the area of the lower basal turn, showing little influence on hearing [*Schuknecht*, pers. commun. 1981].

After the pick perforates the round window membrane, it creates fistulae in the osseous spiral lamina, the limbus spiralis and the cochlear duct. *Schuknecht* describes the importance of creating a fistula in the osseous spiral lamina, in particular, because a fistula in this region cannot be easily closed. In this case, the part of the round window membrane perforated is usually the pars posterior. Immediately after the operation, the runoff of inner ear fluids from the round window membrane is extremely slight.

The following case is an example of Ménière's disease treated by this method.

Subject K.I., a 54-year-old male. Chief complaints: hearing loss in the right ear, tinnitus and dizziness. The patient had complained of hearing loss and tinnitus in his right ear since 1974, followed by dizziness and an aggravation of the cochlear symptoms in September 1978. A vertiginous attack continued for a few days each time, with a total of 4–5 attacks per year. At the time of the first clinical examination, sensorineural hearing loss of 43 dB on average was detected, as well as a positive reaction to both the ABLB and the Metz tests. On examining the vestibular functions, it was observed that the right ear showed canal paresis in the caloric test. X-ray film showed a normal internal auditory meatus.

On January 17, 1979, decompression of the endolymphatic sac was performed on the right ear. After this operation, vertiginous attacks disappeared, while hearing progressively worsened and tinnitus as well as an ache in the back of the head became worse. In September 1981, the right ear showed sensorineural hearing loss of 56 dB on average, and speech discrimination was at the maximum 50%. A feeling of stuffiness in the ear and slight dizziness were experienced by the patient, as a result of which a cochleosacculotomy was performed in November of the same year. The patient mentioned that since the operation, he had not experienced dizziness, and that the tinnitus and ringing in the head had been alleviated. He also said that his head seemed to have become 'lightened'. Hearing deteriorated to a profound temporary deafness after the operation, but was gradually regained; with the exception of the 8,000 Hz range, it returned after 6 weeks almost to the same level as before the operation (fig. 78). Since then, there have been no vertiginous attacks.

Of the various surgical treatments for Ménière's disease which have been devised, decompression of the endolymphatic sac at present is predominant. This method has gained popularity through the fact that fewer vertiginous attacks are experienced after the operation, while hearing is maintained at the preoperative level, achieving a relatively favorable overall result. This treatment is not always feasible, however, since there are some endolymphatic sacs which are either hypoplastic or sealed off. In these cases, cochleosacculotomy is feasible on practically all occasions. It will take many years to

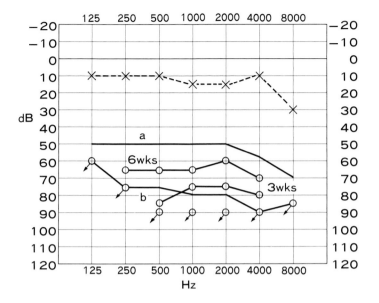

Fig. 78. Changes in hearing after cochlear endolymphatic shunt. a and b show the range of changes in hearing for the past year.

judge the true value of this surgical method, but the patients we have treated describe the postoperative condition of their ears as 'cleared up'. They have remained free from stuffiness of the ear.

Schuknecht [1982] stated that postoperative hearing loss occurs only in the high frequencies. From our experience, young patients with relatively good hearing maintain their hearing after the operation in all frequencies except 8,000 Hz or 4,000 and 8,000 Hz. Aged patients with moderate hearing loss show a tendency to have their hearing deteriorated. It is remarkable that hyperacusis in cochlear Ménière's disease has disappeared in all 3 patients we have treated while hearing is preserved [*Nomura* et al., 1983]. Cochlear endolymphatic shunt is also indicated as a suitable surgical treatment for delayed endolymphatic hydrops where profound hearing loss is recognized. Vertigo can be relieved without the risk of complications.

Singular Neurectomy

It was suggested by *Schuknecht* [1969] that benign paroxysmal positional vertigo (BPPV) is caused by the pathological alteration of the cupula of the posterior ampulla; hence the name cupulolithiasis (fig. 60). As a treatment for BPPV, active exercise is encouraged. In cases of intractable BPPV, a neurectomy of the singular nerve, innervating the posterior ampulla, is performed. This method was first reported by *Gacek* [1974]. Cases reported showed the following symptoms, induced by certain head positions and persisting for 1–12 years: (1) A sensation of vertigo. (2) A latent period of nystagmus between assuming the provocative position and the onset of vertigo. (3) Relatively short duration of vertiginous attack and nystagmus. (4) A rotatory nystagmus lasting for 5–25 s and directed toward the undermost ear. (5) Fatigability on repeated testing. (6) Reproducibility of vertigo, and reversibility of the direction of nystagmus when the patient is returned to the starting position.

Gacek [1974] conducted a singular neurectomy by performing a tympanotomy beforehand. The round window niche is scraped open, and it is important, then, that the entire round window membrane be exposed. As the area attached directly beneath the round window membrane is drilled to 1.5–2 mm deep in an oval shape, the singular nerve appears parallel to the attachment area. The singular nerve is cut off; a pick is inserted from the nearest end of the singular canal to allow sufficient excochleation, and gelfoam is packed tightly into the area where the bone is missing. The operation is completed when the tympanic membrane is returned to the original position. *Gacek* [1978] revised his surgical technique later, however. In the modified technique, he revised the route to the singular nerve from the lateral side of the round window niche to its inferior side. This alteration enables the preservation of the bony margin of the round window niche to a certain degree, thereby reducing cochlear impairment.

Epley [1980] conducted a singular neurectomy after hypotympanotomy. Since the round window membrane lies horizontal, the singular nerve, which is located medially to the membrane, cannot be identified unless observed from below. This operation is difficult when the jugular bulb is situated in a relatively high position or when the singular canal is more or less high. There is some speculation that the jugular bulb and the singular canal are closely related in anatomical location [*Gacek*, 1974].

Complications resulting from neurectomy include sensorineural hearing loss induced by damage to the cochlea, liquorrhea, and impairment of the posterior ampulla. If the drilling to open the round window niche is extended further forward, the cochlear aqueduct and the inferior cochlear vein may be impaired. It has been nearly 8 years since this surgical method was first introduced. As of October 1981, 96 patients in the United States had undergone this surgery. 91% of the patients reported that vertigo disappeared as a result of the operation. 7.3% experienced sensorineural hearing loss [*Gacek*, pers. commun., 1981].

As is apparent from the sectional specimens of the cochlea, that the singular nerve runs medial to the round window membrane and above it. Unless the round window membrane is observed from below, it is impossible to reach the nerve. It should be noted, further, that the space between the nerve and the vestibule is extremely narrow. If the round window is exposed carelessly, the vestibule can easily be damaged. In order to avoid this secondary damage, care must be taken once the singular nerve is exposed (see chapter 7).

References and Selected Reading

1. Brief History of Studies of the Cochlear Window

Békésy, G.V.: The sound pressure difference between the round and the oval windows and the artificial window of labyrinthine fenestration. Acta oto-lar. *35:* 301–315 (1947).

Békésy, G.V.: Experiments in hearing (McGraw-Hill, New York 1960).

Culler, E.; Finch, G.; Girden, E.S.: Function of the round window. Science *78:* 269–270 (1933).

Culler, E.; Finch, G.; Girden, E.: Function of the round window in hearing. Am. J. Physiol. *111:* 416–425 (1935).

Denker, A.; Kahler, O.: Handbuch der Hals-Nasen-Ohrenheilkunde, vol. 6, pp. 458–462 (Springer, Berlin 1926).

Garcia-Ibáñez, L.: Un nuevo sistema audioquirúrgico: la sonoinversión. (nota previa). Revta esp. Oto-neuro-oftal. Neurocirug. *16:* 73–76 (1959).

Gisselsson, L.; Richter, O.: Ein Beitrag zur Frage des Hörvermögens bei Verschluss des runden Fensters. Arch. Ohr.-Nas. KehlkHeilk. *166:* 410–418 (1955).

Goodhill, V.; Holocomb, A.L.; Rehman, I. et al.: Cochlear microphonic measurements in experimental labyrinthine occlusion and fenestration. Laryngoscope *64:* 333–344 (1954).

Groen, J.J.; Hoogland, G.A.: Bone conduction and otosclerosis of the round window. Acta oto-lar. *49:* 206–212 (1958).

Habermann, J.: Zur Pathologie der Taubstummheit und der Fensternischen. Arch. Ohrenheilk. *53:* 52–67 (1901).

Hallpike, C.S.; Scott, P.: Observations on the function of the round window. J. Physiol. *99:* 76–82 (1940).

Hughson, W.; Crowe, S.J.: Function of the round window. An experimental study. J. Am. med. Ass. *96:* 2027–2028 (1931).

Hughson, W.; Crowe, S.J.: Immobilization of the round window membrane: a further experimental study. Ann. Otol. Rhinol. Lar. *41:* 332–348 (1932).

Kirikae, I.: The structure and function of the middle ear (University of Tokyo Press, Tokyo 1960).

Kobrak, H.G.: Round window membrane of the cochlea. Archs Otolar. *49:* 36–47 (1949).

Kobrak, H.G.: The middle ear (University of Chicago Press, Chicago 1959).

Link, R.: Zur Funktion des runden Fensters und des Schalleitungsapparates. Hals-Nas.-Ohrenarzt *33:* 241 (1943).

McNally, W.J.: Puncture of the round window membrane. Experiments on the saccus endolymphaticus. Archs Otolar. *5:* 30–38 (1927).

Oppikofer, E.: Über das Vorkommen von Fett in der runden Fensternische. Z. Ohrenheilk. *75:* 50–65 (1917).

Ranke, O.F.: Discussion remark to Meyer zum Gottesberge: Die Schalleitung im Mittelohr in klinischer Sicht. Z. Lar. Rhinol. Otol. *37:* 366–367 (1958).

Ranke, O.F.; Keidel, W.D.; Weschke, H.G.: Das Hören beim Verschluss des runden Fensters. Z. Lar. Rhinol. Otol. *31:* 467–475 (1952).

Sato, Y.: Surgery for hearing improvement. A. Basic problems. Proc. XVI Gen. Assemb. Jpn. Med. Congr., pp. 603–604 (1963).

Scarpa, A.: De structura fenestrae rotundae auris, et de tympano secundario anatomicae observationes. Apud Societatem Typographicam, Mutinae 1772 (translated and edited by Sellers, L.M., Anson, B.J.). Archs Otolar. *75:* 2–45 (1962).

Sellers, L.M.: The round window – a critical re-evaluation. Laryngoscope *71:* 237–257 (1961).

Simmons, F.B.; Beatty, D.L.: The significance of round-window-recorded cochlear potentials in hearing. Ann. Otol. Rhinol. Lar. *71:* 767–800 (1962).

Stevenson, E.W.: Conduction of sound by a round-window columella. A case resulting in normal hearing. Archs Otolar. *74:* 81–84 (1961).

Tonndorf, J.; Tabor, J.R.: Closure of the cochlear windows. Its effect upon air and bone conduction. Ann. Otol. Rhinol. Lar. *71:* 5–29 (1962).

Weber-Liel: Die Membrana tympani secundaria. Mschr. Ohrenheilk. Lar.-Rhinol. *1:* 8–12 suppl., pp. 8–12 (1876).

Weber-Liel: Weitere anatomische und physicalische Untersuchungen über die Membrana tympani secundaria. Mschr. Ohrenheilk. Lar.-Rhinol. *5:* suppl., pp. 72–76 (1876).

Wever, E.G.; Lawrence, M.: The function of the round window. Ann. Otol. Rhinol. Lar. *57:* 579–589 (1948).

2. Phylogenesis

Burlet, H.M. de: Der perilymphatische Raum des Meerschweinchenohres. Anat. Anz. *53:* 302–315 (1920).

Burlet, H.M. de: Zur vergleichenden Anatomie und Physiologie des perilymphatischen Raumes. Acta oto-lar. *13:* 153–187 (1928/29).

Portmann, A.: Einführung in die vergleichende Morphologie der Wirbeltiere (Schwabe, Basel 1976).

Tumarkin, A.: On the evolution of the auditory perilymphatic system. J. Lar. Otol. *62:* 691–701 (1948).

Turner, R.G.: Physiology and bioacoustics in reptiles; in Popper, Fay, Comparative studies in hearing in vertebrates, pp. 205–237 (Springer, New York 1980).

3. Embryology

Anson, B.J.; Bast, T.H.: The development of the otic capsule in the region of the cochlear fenestra. Ann. Otol. Rhinol. Lar. *62:* 1083–1116 (1953).

Anson, B.J.; Bast, T.H.; Cauldwell, E.W.: The development of the auditory ossicles, the otic capsule and the extracapsular tissue. Ann. Otol. Rhinol. Lar. *57:* 603–632 (1948).

Bast, T.H.: Development of the otic capsule. VI. Histological changes and variations in the growing bony capsule of the vestibule and cochlea. Ann. Otol. Rhinol. Lar. *51:* 343–357 (1942).

Bast, T.H.: Development of the aqueductus cochleae and its contained periotic duct and cochlear vein in human embryos. Ann. Otol. Rhinol. Lar. *55:* 278–297 (1946).

Bast, T.H.; Anson, B.J.: The development of the cochlear fenestra, fossula and secondary tympanic membrane. NWest. Univ. med. School Q. Bull. *25/26:* 344–373 (1952).

Cauldwell, E.W.; Anson, B.J.: Stapes, fissula ante fenestram and associated structures in man. III. From embryos 6.7 to 55 mm in length. Archs Otolar. *36:* 891–925 (1942).

Foley, J.O.: The cytological process involved in the formation of the scalae of the internal ear. Anat. Rec. *49:* 1–14 (1931).

Frick, H.: Über die Aufteilung des Foramen perilymphaticum in der Ontogenese der Säuger. Z. Anat. EntwGesch. *116:* 523–551 (1952).

Frick, H.: Über die Entwicklung der Schneckenfensternische (Fossula fenestrae rotundae) beim Menschen. Arch. Ohr.-Nas. KehlkHeilk. *162:* 520–534 (1953).

Streeter, G.L.: The development of the scala tympani, scala vestibuli and periotic cistern in human embryo. Am. J. Anat. *21:* 299–320 (1917).

Streeter, G.L.: The factors involved in the excavation of the cavities in the cartilaginous capsule of the ear in the human embryo. Am. J. Anat. *22:* 1–25 (1917).

Streeter, G.L.: The histogenesis and growth of the otic capsule and its contained periotic tissue-spaces in the human embryo. Contr. Embryol. *7:* 5 (1918).

Waltner, J.G.: Development of the cochlear aqueduct and the round window membrane in human embryo. Archs Otolar. *42:* 239–252 (1945).

Waltner, J.G.: Barrier membrane of the cochlear aqueduct. Histologic studies on the patency of the cochlear aqueduct. Archs Otolar. *47:* 656–669 (1948).

4. Round Window Niche and Round Window Membrane

5. Round Window Membrane (Shape and Structure)

Ainsworth, S.K.; Karnovsky, M.J.: An ultrastructural staining method for enhancing the size and electron capacity of ferritin in thin sections. J. Histochem. Cytochem. *20:* 225–229 (1972).

Alexander, G.: Das Labyrinthpigment des Menschen und der höheren Säugethiere. Arch. mikrosk. Anat. EntwGesch. *58:* 134–181 (1901).

Andrzejewski, C.: Über die feinere Histologie des Nervengewebes in der Membrana tympani, Membrana tympani secundaria und Mucosa der Paukenhöhle von Mensch und Hund. Z. Zellforsch. *39:* 447–469 (1954).

Anson, B.J.: Stapedial, capsular and labyrinthine anatomy in relation to otologic surgery. Ann. Otol. Rhinol. Lar. *70:* 607–631 (1961).

Anson, B.J.; Donaldson, J.A.: Surgical anatomy of the temporal bone (Saunders, Philadelphia 1981).

Anson, B.J.; Donaldson, J.A.; Warpeha, R.L., et al.: A critical appraisal of the anatomy of the perilymphatic system in man. Laryngoscope *74:* 945–966 (1964).

Arnold, W.: Die Bedeutung des subepithelialen Raumes der Mittelohrschleimhaut. Arch. klin. exp. Ohr.-Nas.-KehlkHeilk. *198:* 262–280 (1971).

Arnold, W.; Ilberg, C.: Die Verbindung zwischen Liquor cerebrospinalis und dem Lymphsystem der Mittelohrschleimhaut. Arch. klin. exp. Ohr.-Nas.-KehlkHeilk. *199:* 453–457 (1971).

Arnold, W.; Ilberg, C.: Neue Aspekte zur Morphologie und Funktion des runden Fensters. Z. Lar. Rhinol. Otol. *51:* 390–399 (1972).

Axelsson, A.: The vascular anatomy of the cochlea in the guinea pig and in man. Acta oto-lar. *243:* suppl., pp. 5–134 (1968).

Bast, T.H.; Anson, B.J.: The temporal bone and the ear (Thomas, Springfield, 1949).

Bast, T.H.; Anson, B.J.: The development of the cochlear fenestra, fossula and secondary tympanic membrane. NWest. Univ. Med. School Q. Bull. *25/26:* 344–373 (1952).

Beck, C.; Bader, J.: Ein Beitrag zur feineren Anatomie des menschlichen Innenohres. Zusammengefasst dargestellt in einem neuen Labyrinthmodell. Arch. Ohr.-Nas.-KehlkHeilk. *181:* 245–267 (1963).

Bellucci, R.J.; Fisher, E.G.; Rhodin, J.: Ultrastructure of the round window membrane. Laryngoscope *82:* 1021–1026 (1972).

Bennett, M.V.L.: Function of electrotonic junctions in embryonic and adult tissue. Fed. Proc. *32:* 65–75 (1973).

Brady, D.R.; Pearce, J.P.; Juhn, S.K.: Permeability of round window membrane to ^{22}Na or RISA. Archs Oto-Rhino-Lar. *214:* 183–184 (1976).

Branton, D.: Fracture faces of frozen membranes. Proc. nat. Acad. Sci. USA *55:* 1048–1056 (1966).

Breuninger, H.; Giebel, W.: Untersuchungen über die Durchgängigkeit der Membran des runden Fensters für Tetracycline. Archs Oto-Rhino-Lar. *210:* 362 (1975).

Carpenter, A.M.; Goycoolea, M.V.: Morphometry of round window changes after Eustachian tube obstruction. Meet. Ass. for Research in Oto-Laryngology, St. Petersburg, Fla. 1979.

Caspar, D.L.D.; Goodenough, D.A.; Makowski, L., et al.: Gap junction structures. 1. Correlated electron microscopy and X-ray diffraction. J. Cell Biol. *74:* 605–628 (1977).

Claude, P.; Goodenough, D.A.: Fracture faces of zonulae occludentes from 'tight and leaky' epithelia. J. Cell Biol. *58:* 390–400 (1973).

Dean, L.W.; Wolff, D.: Pathology and routes of infection in labyrinthitis secondary to middle ear otitis. Ann. Otol. Rhinol. Lar. *43:* 702–717 (1934).

Donaldson, J.A.: Fossula of the cochlear fenestra. Archs Otolar. *88:* 124–130 (1968).

Franke, K.: Elektronenmikroskopische Befunde der Membran des runden Fensters. Archs Oto-Rhino-Lar. *216:* 522 (1977a).

Franke, K.: Freeze-fracture aspects of the junctional complexes in the round window membrane. Archs Oto-Rhino-Lar. *217:* 331–337 (1977b).

Franke, K.: Fine structure of the tissue lining the cochlear perilymphatic space against the bony labyrinthine capsule. Archs Oto-Rhino-Lar. *222:* 161–167 (1979).

Frick, H.: Über die Entwicklung der Schneckenfensternische (Fossula fenestrae rotundae) beim Menschen. Arch. Ohr-Nas.-KehlkHeilk. *162:* 520–534 (1953).

Friend, D.S.; Gilula, N.B.: Variation in tight and gap junctions in mammalian tissues. J. Cell. Biol. *53:* 758–776 (1972).

Galle, E.; Siegel, G.: The transport of radioactive labelled sodium ions at the round window. Acta oto-lar. *79:* 108–110 (1975).

Gillespie, C.A.; Swanson, G.C.; Johnson, C.M. et al.: Inner ear lidocaine concentrations following iontophoresis. Laryngoscope *90:* 1845–1851 (1980).

Goycoolea, M.V.; Paparella, M.M.; Goldberg, B., et al.: Permeability of the middle ear to staphylococcal pyrogenic exotoxin in otitis media. Int. J. pediat Otorhinolar. *1:* 301–308 (1980a).

Goycoolea, M.V.; Paparella, M.M.; Goldberg, B., et al.: Permeability of the round window membrane in otitis media. Archs Otolar. *106:* 430–433 (1980b).

Goycoolea, M.V.; Paparella, M.M.; Juhn, S.K., et al.: Oval and round window changes in otitis media: an experimental study in the cat. Surg. Forum *29:* 578–580 (1978).

Graham, R.C.; Karnovsky, M.J.: The early stages of absorption of injected horseradish peroxidase in the proximal tubules of mouse kidney. Ultrastructural cytochemistry by a new technique. J. Histochem. Cytochem. *14:* 291–302 (1966).

Gussen, R.: Round window niche melanocytes and webby tissue. Archs Otolar. *104:* 662–668 (1978).

Harty, M.: The secondary tympanic membrane and annular ligament. Z. mikrosk.-anat. Forsch. *70:* 484–489 (1963).

Hata, A.: Permeability of the round window membrane, with special regard to kanamycin ototoxicity. Pract. Otol., Kyoto *60:* 429–436 (1968).

Hattori, Y.; Yuge, K.: Electron microscopic studies of the tympanic membrane and the round window membrane. Otol. Fukuoka *25:* 1115–1138 (1979).

Hayashi, T.; Nagai, Y.: Separation of the α chains of type I and III collagens by SDS-polyacrylamide gel electrophoresis. J. Biochem. *86:* 453–459 (1979).

Helmholtz, H.L.F.: cited by Wever, E.G.; Lawrence, M.: Physiological acoustics (Princeton University Press, Princeton 1954).

Höft, J.: Elektronenmikroskopische Untersuchungen über die Durchlässigkeit der Membran des runden Fensters beim Meerschweinchen. Arch. klin. exp. Ohr.-Nas.-KehlkHeilk. *191:* 539–540 (1968).

Höft, J.: Die Permeabilität und die Beeinflussung der Permeabilität der Membran des runden Fensters durch Pantocain (Tetracain). Arch. klin. exp. Ohr.-Nas.-KehlkHeilk *193:* 128–137 (1969).

Kaupp, H.; Giebel, W.: Distribution of marked perilymph to the subarachnoidal space. Archs Oto-Rhino-Lar. *229:* 245–253 (1980).

Kawabata, I.; Ishii, H.: Fiber arrangement in the tympanic membrane. Scanning electron microscope observations. Acta oto-lar. *72:* 243–254 (1971).

Kawabata, I.; Paparella, M.M.: Fine structure of the round window membrane. Ann. Otol. Rhinol. Lar. *80:* 13–26 (1971).

Keith, A.; cited by Wever, E.G.; Lawrence, M.: Physiological acoustics (Princeton University Press, Princeton 1954).

Khanna, S.M.; Tonndorf, J.: The vibratory pattern of the round window in cats. J. acoust. Soc. Am. *50:* 1475–1483 (1971).

Kirikae, I.: The structure and function of the middle ear (University of Tokyo Press, Tokyo 1960).

Kobrak, H.G.: Round window membrane of the cochlea. Archs Otolar. *49:* 36–47 (1949).

Kölliker, A.: cited by Schaefer, K.L.; Giesswein, M.

Lim, D.J.: Human tympanic membrane. An ultrastructural observation. Acta oto-lar. *70:* 176–186 (1970).

Lim, D.J.: Functional morphology of the lining membrane of the middle ear and Eustachian tube. Ann. Otol. Rhinol. Lar. *83:* suppl. 11, pp. 5–26 (1974).

Link, R.: Beitrag zur Histologie der Membran des runden Fensters. Z. Lar. Rhinol. Otol. *32:* 295–302 (1942).

McNutt, N.S.; Weinstein, R.S.: Membrane ultrastructure at mammalian intercellular junctions. Prog. Biophys. molec. Biol. *26:* 45–101 (1973).

Miriszlai, E.; Benedeczky, I.; Csapó, S., et al.: The ultrastructure of the round window membrane of the cat. ORL *40:* 111–119 (1978).

Miriszlai, E.; Benedeczky, I.; Horváth, K.; Köllner, P.: Ultrastructural organization of the round window membrane in the infant human middle ear. ORL *45:* 29–38 (1983).

Murakami, T.; Yamamoto, K.; Itoshima, T.; Irino, S.: Modified tannin-osmium conductive staining method for non-coated scanning electron microscope specimens. Its application to microdissection scanning electronmicroscopy of the spleen. Arch. histol. jap. *40:* 35–40 (1977).

Nakai, Y.; Kaneko, M.: Round window membrane. Submicroscopic structure and permeability. Pract. Otol., Kyoto *68:* 223–232 (1975).

Nomura, Y.: A needle otoscope. Acta oto-lar. *93:* 73–79 (1982a).

Nomura, Y.: Effective photography in otolaryngology – head and neck surgery: endoscopic photography of the middle ear. Otolar. Head Neck Surg. *90:* 395–398 (1982b).

Ogura, Y.: A holographic study of the eardrum vibration. Otolaryngology, Tokyo *46:* 83–88 (1974).

Ogura, Y.; Kimura, Y.; Uyemura, T., et al.: Application of holography to the study of hearing. Analysis of the eardrum vibration. Okayama I Z *86:* 215–219 (1974).

Ogura, Y.; Masuda, Y.; Miki, M., et al.: A holographic study of the human skull vibration. Audiol. Jap. *19:* 163–167 (1976).

Orsuláková, A.; Stupp, H.F.: Experimentelle pH-Veränderungen im Mittelohr und ihre Wirkung auf das Innenohr. Archs Oto-Rhino-Lar. *209:* 23–31, (1975).

Panse: Die Schwerhörigkeit durch Starrheit der Paukenfenster, 1897; cited by Denker, A.; Kahler, O.: Die Krankheiten des Gehörorgans (1926).

Paparella, M.M.: Insidious labyrinthine changes in otitis media. Acta oto-lar. *92:* 513–520 (1981).

Rauch, S.: Quantitative Angaben über die Durchlässigkeit der 'Membranen' des runden und ovalen Fensters der Cochlea. Practica oto-rhino-lar. *28:* 389–397 (1966).

Rhodes, T.: Round window membrane permeability to horseradish peroxidase: an electron microscopy study: thesis University of Minnesota Graduate School, Minneapolis (1980).

Richardson, T.L.; Ishiyama, E.; Keels, E.W.: Submicroscopic studies of the round window membrane. Acta oto-lar. *71:* 9–21 (1971).

Saijo, S.; Kimura, R.S.: Distribution of horseradish peroxidase in the inner ear after injection into the middle ear cavity. Abstr. Research Forum, ARO, 1981.

Sawashima, M.: Special situation and areas of the tympanic membrane, the oval and the round window in the human temporal bone. J. Otolaryngol. Jpn. *61:* 247–251 (1958).

Schaefer, K.L.; Giesswein, M.: Physiologie des Ohres. 1. Physiologie des äusseren und mittleren Ohres und der Schnecke; in Denker, Kahler, Handbuch der Hals-Nasen-Ohren-Heilkunde, vol. VI: Die Krankheiten des Gehörorgans, vol. 1, pp. 389–518 (1926).

Schicker, S.: Das runde Fenster. Laryngologie *36:* 149–153 (1957).

Sekine, M.; Sasahara, K.; Kojima, T., et al.: High-performance liquid chromatographic method for determination of cefmetazole in human serum. Antimicrob. Agents Chemother. *21:* 740–743 (1982).

Simionescu, M.; Simionescu, N.; Palade, G.E.: Segmental differentiations of cell junctions in the vascular epithelium. Arteries and veins. J. Cell Biol. *68:* 705–723 (1975).

Smith, B.M.; Myers, M.G.: The penetration of gentamicin and neomycin into perilymph across the round window membrane. Otolar. Head Neck Surg. *87:* 888–891 (1979).

Staehelin, L.A.: Structure and function of intercellular junctions. Int. Rev. Cytol. *39:* 191–283 (1974).

Stecker, R.H.; Cody, T.R.: Iontophoresis of [22]Na and ^{131}I into the inner ear. Archs Otolar. *83:* 213–217 (1966).

Stewart, T.J.; Belal, A.: Surgical anatomy and pathology of the round window. Clin. Otolaryngol. *6:* 45–62 (1981).

Su, W.J.; Marion, M.S.; Hinojosa, R.; Matz, G.J.: Anatomical measurements of the cochlear aqueduct, round window membrane, round window niche, and facial recess. Laryngoscope *92:* 483–486 (1982).

Tanaka, K.; Motomura, S.: Permeability of the labyrinthine windows in guinea pigs. Archs Oto-Rhino-Lar. *233:* 67–75 (1981).

Tröltsch, A. v.: cited by Schaefer, K.L.; Giesswein, M.

Wever, E.G.; Lawrence, M.: Physiological acoustics (Princeton University Press, Princeton 1954).

Werner, C.I.F.: Das Gehörorgan der Wirbeltiere und des Menschen. Beispiel für eine vergleichende Morphologie der Lagebeziehungen (Thieme, Leipzig 1960).

Wolff, D.: Melanin in the inner ear. Archs Otolar. *14:* 195–211 (1931).

6. Pathology

Adkins, W.Y., Jr.; Gussen, R.: Oval window absence, bony closure of round window, and inner ear anomaly. Laryngoscope *84:* 1210–1224 (1974).

Altmann, F.: The ear in severe malformations of the head: a discussion of the formal and causal genetic factors involved. Archs Otolar. *66:* 7–25 (1957).

Belal, A., Jr.: Pathology of vascular sensorineural hearing impairment. Laryngoscope *90:* 1831–1839 (1980).

Dean, L.W.; Wolff, D.: Pathology and routes of infection in labyrinthitis secondary to middle ear otitis. Ann. Otol. Rhinol. Lar. *43:* 702–717 (1934).

Fleischer, K.: Otosclerose am runden Fenster. Z. Lar. Rhinol. Otol. *41:* 447–453 (1962).

Goycoolea, M.V.; Paparella, M.M.; Juhn, S.K., et al.: Oval and round window changes in otitis media. Potential pathways between middle and inner ear. Laryngoscope *90:* 1387–1391 (1980).

Guild, S.R.: Histologic otosclerosis. Ann. Otol. Rhinol. Lar. *53:* 246–266 (1944).

Guild, S.R.: Incidence, location and extent of otosclerotic lesions. Archs Otolar. *52:* 848–852 (1950).

Harada, T.; Hiraide, F.; Nomura, Y.: Histological otosclerosis in a Japanese. A case with multiple foci and crista neglecta. ANL *2:* 29–36 (1975).

Harada, T.; Sando, I.: Temporal bone histopathologic findings in Down's syndrome. Archs Otolar. *107:* 96–103 (1981).

Igarashi, M.; Schuknecht, H.F.: Pneumococcic otitis media, meningitis and labyrinthitis. Archs Otolar. *76:* 126–130 (1962).

Kimura, R.; Perlman, H.B.: Arterial obstruction of the labyrinth. I. Cochlear changes. Ann. Otol. Rhinol. Lar. *67:* 5–24 (1958).

Lindsay, J.R.: Histopathology of otosclerosis. Archs Otolar. *97:* 24–29 (1973).

Lindsay, J.R.; Hemenway, W.G.: Occlusion of the round window by otosclerosis. Laryngoscope *64:* 10–19 (1954).

Meyerhoff, W.L.; Shea, D.A.; Giebink, G.S.: Experimental pneumococcal otitis media: a histopathologic study. Otolar. Head Neck Surg. *88:* 606–612 (1980).

Nager, F.R.: Die pathologische Anatomie des endemisch-kretinisch erkrankten Gehörorgans; in Denker, Kahler, Handbuch der Hals-Nasen-Ohren-Heilkunde, vol. VI: Die Krankheiten des Gehörorgans, vol. 1, p. 621 (1926).

Nager, F.R.; Fraser, J.S.: On bone formation in the scala tympani of otosclerotics. J. Lar. Otol. *53:* 173–180 (1938).

Nomura, Y.; Hiraide, F.: Congenital anomalies of the inner ear. Audiol. Jap. *15:* 165–172 (1972).

Nomura, Y.; Tsuchida, M.; Mori, S., et al.: Deafness in cryoglobulinemia. Ann. Otol. Rhinol. Lar. *91:* 250–255 (1982).

Nylén, B.: Histopathological investigations on the localization, number, activity and extent of otosclerotic foci. J. Lar. Otol. *63:* 321–327 (1949).

Saito, Y.; Kitahara, M.; Kitajima, K., et al.: Meningogenic meningitis. Pract. Otol., Kyoto *74:* suppl. 5, pp. 2341–2345 (1981).

Stewart, T.J.; Belal, A.: Surgical anatomy and pathology of the round window. Clin. Otolaryngol. *6:* 45–62 (1981).

7. Anatomy of the Circumference of the Round Window

Ahlén, G.: On the connection between cerebrospinal and intralabyrinthine pressure and pressure variations in the inner ear. Acta oto-lar. *35:* 251–257 (1947).

Allan, A.L.: Pneumatization of the temporal bone. Ann. Otol. Rhinol. Lar. *78:* 49–64 (1969).

Altman, F.; Waltner, J.G.: The circulation of the labyrinthine fluids. Experimental investigations in rabbits. Ann. Otol. Rhinol. Lar. *56:* 684–708 (1947).

Anson, B.J.; Donaldson, J.A.; Warpeha, R.L., et al.: A critical appraisal of the anatomy of the perilymphatic system in man. Laryngoscope *74:* 945–966 (1964).

Anson, B.J.; Donaldson, J.A.; Warpeha, R.L., et al.: The vestibular and cochlear aqueducts: their variational anatomy in the adult human ear. Laryngoscope *75:* 1203–1223 (1965).

Arnvig, J.: Transitory decrease of hearing after lumbar puncture. A personal experience which throws some light on the function of the aqueducts of the cochleae. Acta oto-lar. *56:* 699–705 (1963).

Bergström, B.: Morphology of the vestibular nerve. II. The number of myelinated vestibular nerve fibers in man of various ages. Acta oto-lar. *76:* 173–179 (1973).

Bergström, B.: Morphology of the vestibular nerve. III. Analysis of the calibers of the myelinated vestibular nerve fibers in man of various ages. Acta oto-lar. *76:* 331–338 (1973).

Dorph, S.; Jensèn, J.; Oigaard, A.: Visualization of canaliculus cochleae by multitomographic tomography. Archs Otolar. *98:* 121–123 (1973).

Epley, J.M.: Singular neurectomy: hypotympanotomy approach. Otolar. Head Neck Surg. *88:* 304–309 (1980).

Farrior, J.B.; Endicott, J.N.: Congenital mixed deafness: cerebrospinal fluid otorrhea. Ablation of the aqueduct of the cochlea. Laryngoscope *81:* 684–699 (1971).

Gacek, R.R.: The maucla neglecta in the feline species. J. comp. Neurol. *116:* 317–323 (1961).

Graham, M.D.: The jugular bulb. Its anatomic and clinical considerations in contemporary otology. Laryngoscope *87:* 105–125 (1977).

Harada, T.; Sando, I.; Myers, E.N.: Microfissure in the oval window area. Ann. Otol. Rhinol. Lar. *90:* 174–180 (1981).

Karbowski, B.: Vergleichend anatomische Studien über den Aquaeductus cochleae und über seine Beziehungen zum Subarachnoidealraum des Gehirns. Mschr. Ohrenheilk. Lar.-Rhinol. *64:* 687–715 (1930).

Kelemen, G.; Denia La Fuente, A.; Olivares, F.P.: The cochlear aqueduct, structural considerations. Laryngoscope *89:* 639–645 (1979).

Kerth, J.D.; Allen, G.W.: Comparison of the perilymphatic and cerebrospinal fluid pressures. Archs Otolar. *77:* 581–585 (1963).

Meurman, Y.: Zur Anatomie des Aquaeductus Cochleae nebst einigen Bemerkungen über dessen Physiologie. Acta Soc. Med. fenn. 'Duodecim' *13:* ser. B, fasc. 1 (1930).

Montandon, P.; Gacek, R.R.; Kimura, R.S.: Crista neglecta in the cat and human. Ann. Otol. Rhinol. Lar. *79:* 105–112 (1970).

Okano, Y.; Myers, E.N.; Dickson, D.R.: Microfissure between the round window niche and posterior canal ampulla. Ann. Otol. Rhinol. Lar. *86:* 49–57 (1977).

Okano, Y.; Sando, I.; Myers, E.N.: Branch of the singular nerve (posterior ampullary nerve) in the otic capsule. Ann. Otol. Rhinol. Lar. *89:* 13–19 (1980).

Oyerton, S.B.; Ritter, F.N.: A high placed jugular bulb in the middle ear: a clinical and temporal bone study. Laryngoscope *83:* 1986–1991 (1973).

Palva, T.: Cochlear aqueduct in infants. Acta oto-lar. *70:* 83–94 (1970).

Palva, T.; Dammert, K.: Human cochlear aqueduct. Acta oto-lar. *246:* suppl., pp. 1–58 (1969).

Rask-Andersen, H.; Stahle, J.; Wilbrand, H.: Human cochlear aqueduct and its accessory canals. Ann. Otol. Rhinol. Lar. *86:* suppl. 42, pp. 1–16 (1977).

Ritter, F.N.; Lawrence, M.: A histological and experimental study of cochlear aqueduct patency in the adult human. Laryngoscope *75:* 1224–1233 (1965).

Waltner, J.G.: Histogenesis of corpora amylacea of the cochlear aqueduct, the internal auditory meatus and the associated cranial nerves. Archs Otolar. *45:* 619–631 (1947).

Waltner, J.G.: Barrier membrane of the cochlear aqueduct. Histologic studies on the patency of the cochlear aqueduct. Archs Otolar. *47:* 656–669 (1948).

Wlodyka, J.: Studies on cochlear aqueduct patency. Ann. Otol. Rhinol. Lar. *87:* 22–28 (1978).

8. Ear Diseases Pertaining to the Round Window
Drug-Induced Hearing Loss

Arnold, W.; Vosteen, K.H.: Die Reaktion der Mittelohrschleimhaut bei Tubenverschluss. Acta oto-lar. *330:* suppl., pp. 48–63 (1975).

Bortnick, E.; Proud, G.O.: Experimental absorption of fluids from the middle ear. Archs Otolar. *81:* 237–242 (1965).

Brady, D.R.; Pearce, J.P.; Juhn, S.K.: Permeability of round window membrane to ^{22}Na or RISA. Archs Oto-Rhino-Lar. *214:* 183–184 (1976).

Breuninger, H.; Giebel, W.; Haug, H.P.: Über das Eindringen von tympanal appliziertem Tetracyclin in das Innenohr des Meerschweinchens. Archs Oto-Rhino-Lar. *216:* 523–524 (1977).

Brummett, R.E.; Harris, R.F.; Lindgren, J.A.: Detection of ototoxicity from drugs applied topically to the middle ear space. Laryngoscope *86:* 1177–1187 (1976).

Fairbanks, D.N.F.: Otic topical agents. Otolar. Head Neck Surg. *88:* 327–331 (1980).

Fowler, E.P., Jr.; Forbes, T.W.: End-organ deafness in dogs due to application of certain chemicals to the round window membrane. Ann. Otol. Rhinol. Lar. *45:* 859–864 (1936).

Galle, E.; Siegel, G.: The transport of radioactive labelled sodium ions at the round window. Acta oto-lar. *79:* 108–110 (1975).

Goycoolea, M.V.; Paparella, M.M.; Goldberg, B.: Permeability of the middle ear to staphylococcal pyrogenic exotoxin in otitis media. Int. J. pediat. Otorhinolar. *1:* 301–308 (1980a).

Goycoolea, M.V.; Paparella, M.M.; Goldberg, B., et al.: Permeability of round window membrane in otitis media. Archs Otolar. *106:* 430–433 (1980b).

Goycoolea, M.V.; Paparella, M.M.; Juhn, S.K., et al.: Oval and round window changes in otitis media. Potential pathways between middle and inner ear. Laryngoscope *90:* 1387–1391 (1980c).

Harris, R.; Brown, R.: The ototoxicity of topically applied neomycin. 18th Annu. Meet. Committee for Research of the American Association of Otolaryngology, 1974.

Kohonen, A.; Tarkkanen, J.: Cochlear damage from ototoxic antibiotics by intratympanic application. Acta oto-lar. *68:* 90–97 (1969).

Lindsay, J.R.; Proctor, L.R.; Work, W.P.: Histopathologic inner ear changes in deafness due to neomycin in a human. Laryngoscope *70:* 382–392 (1960).

Lundquist, G.; Wersäll, J.: Site of action of ototoxic antibiotics after local and general administration; in Vestibular function on earth and in space, pp. 267–274 (Pergamon Press, New York 1970).

Mittelman, H.: Ototoxicity of 'ototopical' antibiotics: past, present, and future. Trans. Am. Acad. Ophthal. Oto-lar. *76:* 1432–1443 (1972).

Morizono, T.; Johnstone, B.M.: Ototoxicity of topically applied gentamicin using a statistical analysis of electrophysiological measurement. Acta oto-lar. *80:* 389–393 (1975).

Nakai, Y.; Yamamoto, K.; Igarashi, M.: Ototoxicity of topically applied antibiotics in guinea pigs and squirrel monkeys. Audiol. Jap. *17:* 190–197 (1974).

Paparella, M.M.; Brady, D.R.; Hoel, R.: Sensori-neural hearing loss in chronic otitis media and mastoiditis. Trans. Am. Acad. Ophthal. Oto-lar. *74:* 108–115 (1970).

Paparella, M.M.; Sugiura, S.: The pathology of suppurative labyrinthitis. Ann. Otol. Rhinol. Lar. *76:* 554–586 (1967).

Patterson, W.C.; Gulick, W.L.: The effects of chloramphenicol upon the electrical activity of the ear. Ann. Otol. Rhinol. Lar. *72:* 50–55 (1963).

Proud, G.O.; Mittelman, H.; Seiden, G.D.: Ototoxicity of topically applied chloramphenicol. Archs Otolar. *87:* 580–587 (1968).

Rahm, W.E., Jr.; Strother, W.F.; Gulick, W.L., et al.: The effects of topical anesthetics upon the ear. Ann. Otol. Rhinol. Lar. *68:* 1037–1046 (1959).

Rahm, W.E., Jr.; Strother, W.F.; Gulick, W.L., et al.: The effects of anesthetics upon the ear. II. Procaine hydrochloride. Ann. Otol. Rhinol. Lar. *69:* 969–975 (1960).

Rahm, W.E., Jr.; Strother, W.F.; Gulick, W.L., et al.: The effects of anesthetics upon the ear. III. Tetracaine hydrochloride. Ann. Otol. Rhinol. Lar. *70:* 403–409 (1961).

Riskaer, N.; Christensen, E.; Petersen, P.V., et al.: The ototoxicity of neomycin. Experimental investigations. Acta oto-lar. *46:* 137–152 (1956).

Smith, B.M.; Myers, M.G.: The penetration of gentamycin and neomycin into perilymph across the round window membrane. Otolar. Head Neck Surg. *87:* 888–891 (1979).

Round Window Membrane Rupture (see chapt. 7)

Ahlén, G.: On the connection between cerebrospinal and intralabyrinthine pressure and pressure variations in the inner ear. Acta oto-lar. *35:* 251–257 (1947).

Allen, G.W.; Habibi, M.: The effect of increasing the cerebrospinal fluid pressure upon the cochlear microphonics. Laryngoscope *72:* 423–434 (1962).

Althaus, S.R.: Perilymph fistulas. Laryngoscope *91:* 538–562 (1981).

Althaus, S.R.; House, H.P.: Long-term results of perilymph fistula repair. Laryngoscope *83:* 1502–1509 (1973).

Arenberg, K.; May, M.; Stroud, M.H.: Perilymphatic fistula: an unusual cause of Ménière's syndrome in a prepubertal child. Laryngoscope *84:* 243–246 (1974).

Arnold, W.J.: Role of perilymph in the early stage of serous otitis. Ann. Otol. Rhinol. Lar. *85:* suppl. 25, pp. 73–80 (1976).

Axelsson, A.; Hallén, O.; Miller, J.M., et al.: Experimentally induced round window membrane lesions. Acta oto-lar. *84:* 1–11 (1977).

Beentjes, B.I.J.: The cochlear aqueduct and pressure of cerebrospinal and endolabyrinthine fluids. Acta oto-lar. *73:* 112–120 (1972).

Boeninghaus, J.: Operationsindikation bei Fensterruptur und Hörsturz. Lar. Rhinol. *60:* 49–52 (1981).

Douek, E.: Perilymph fistula. J. Lar. Otol. *89:* 123–130 (1975).

Dysart, B.R.: Spontaneous cerebrospinal otorrhea. Laryngoscope *69:* 935–939 (1959).

Facer, G.W.; Farrell, K.H.; Cody, D.T.R.: Spontaneous perilymph fistula. A medical emergency. Mayo Clin. Proc. *48:* 203–206 (1973).

Fee, G.A.: Traumatic perilymphatic fistulas. Archs Otolar. *88:* 477–480 (1968).

Fernandes, C.M.C.: Labyrinthine membrane rupture: a cause of post-traumatic vertigo. S. Afr. J. Surg. *15:* 71–74 (1977).

Freeman, P.; Tonkin, J.; Edmonds, C.: Rupture of the round window membrane in inner ear barotrauma. Archs Otolar. *99:* 437–442 (1974).

Fukaya, T.; Nomura, Y.: Experimental round window membrane rupture. Electrophysiological consequences in guinea pigs. Audiol. Jap. *24:* 152–155 (1981).

Ganzer, U.G.W.; Arnold, W.: Das Innenohrhörvermögen beim chronischen Seromukotympanon. Lar. Rhinol. *56:* 850–859 (1977).

Goodhill, V.: Sudden deafness and round window rupture. Laryngoscope *81:* 1462–1474 (1971).

Goodhill, V.: Labyrinthine membrane ruptures in sudden sensorineural hearing loss. Proc. R. Soc. Med. *69:* 565–572 (1976).

Goodhill, V.: Leaking labyrinth lesions, deafness, tinnitus and dizziness. Ann. Otol. Rhinol. Lar. *90:* 99–106 (1981).

Gordon, A.G.: Perilymph fistula: a cause of auditory, vestibular, neurological and psychiatric disorders. Med. Hypoth. *2:* 125 (1976).

Grundfast, K.M.; Bluestone, C.D.: Sudden or fluctuating hearing loss and vertigo in children due to perilymph fistula. Ann. Otol. Rhinol. Lar. *87:* 761–771 (1978).

Gyo, K.; Tadokoro, H.; Yanagihara, N.: Clinical findings in labyrinthine window rupture. J. Otolar. Jap. *84:* 975–982 (1981).

Gyo, K.; Yanagihara, H.; Aritomo, H., et al.: Healing process of the experimentally produced round-window-membrane perforation. Pract. Otol., Kyoto *73:* 1543–1549 (1980).

Harker, L.A.; Norante, J.D.; Ryu, J.H.: Experimental rupture of the round window membrane. Trans. Am. Acad. Ophthal. Oto-lar. *78:* 448–452 (1974).

Harrison, W.H.; Shambaugh, G.E.; Derlacki, E.L., et al.: The perilymph fistula problem. Laryngoscope *80:* 1000–1007 (1963).

Healy, G.B.; Friedman, J.M.; Ditroia, J.: Ataxia and hearing loss secondary to perilymphatic fistula. Pediatrics *61:* 238–241 (1978).

Holden, H.; Schuknecht, H.: Distribution pattern of blood in the inner ear following spontaneous subarachnoid haemorrhage. J. Lar. Otol. *82:* 321–329 (1968).

Ivarsson, A.; Pedersen, K.: Volume-pressure properties of round and oval windows. A quantitative study on human temporal bone. Acta oto-lar. *84:* 38–43 (1977).

Kerth, J.D.; Allen, G.W.: Comparison of the perilymphatic and cerebrospinal fluid pressures. Archs Otolar. *77:* 581–585 (1963).

Kline, O.R.: Spontaneous cerebrospinal otorrhea. Archs Otolar. *18:* 34–39 (1933).

Knight, N.J.: Severe sensorineural deafness in children due to perforation of the round window membrane. Lancet *ii:* 1003–1005 (1977).

Kobrak, H.: Untersuchungen über Zusammenhang zwischen Hirndruck und Labyrinthdruck. Passow-Schaefer Beitr. prakt. theor. Hals- Nas.- Ohrenheilk. *31:* 216–240 (1934).

Kohut, R.J.; Waldorf, R.A.; Haenel, J.L., et al.: Minute perilymphatic fistulas. Vertigo and Hennebert's sign without hearing loss. Ann. Otol. Rhinol. Lar. *88:* 153–159 (1979).

Kramer, S.A.; Yanagisawa, E.; Smith, H.W.: Spontaneous cerebrospinal fluid otorrhea simulating serous otitis media. Laryngoscope *81:* 1083–1089 (1971).

Lamkin, R.; Axelsson, A.; McPherson, P., et al.: Experimental aural barotrauma. Electrophysiological and morphological findings. Acta oto-lar. *335:* suppl., pp. 1–24 (1975).

Magnuson, B.: On the origin of the high negative pressure in the middle ear space. Am. J. Otolar. *2:* 1–12 (1981).

McClure, A.; Lycett, P.: Effect of round window removal on auditory thresholds in cats. J. Otolar. *9:* 215–221 (1980).

McCormick, J.G.; Wever, E.G.; Harrill, J.A., et al.: Anatomical and physiological adaptations of marine mammals for the prevention of diving induced middle ear barotrauma and round window fistula. J. acoust. Soc. Am. *58:* S88(A) (1975).

Meurman, Y.: Observations on some pressure phenomena accompanying artificial labyrinthine fistula. Acta oto-lar. *13:* 552–571 (1929).

Miriszlai, E.; Sándor, P.: Investigations on the critical perilymphatic pressure value causing round window membrane rupture in anesthetized cats. Acta oto-lar. *89:* 323–329 (1980).

Moscovitch, D.H.; Gannon, R.P.; Laszlo, C.A.: Perilymph displacement by cerebrospinal fluid in the cochlea. Ann. Otol. Rhinol. Lar. *82:* 53–61 (1973).

Myers, P.W.: Jugular vein compression and elevation of perilymphatic fluid pressure. Archs Otolar. *98:* 314–315 (1973).

Palva, T.: Cochlear aqueduct in infants. Acta oto-lar. *70:* 83–94 (1970).

Palva, T.; Dammert, K.: Human cochlear aqueduct. Acta oto-lar. *246:* suppl., pp. 1–58 (1969).

Pulec, J.L.: Perilymph fistula. Laryngoscope *79:* 868–886 (1969).

Pullen, F.W., II; Rosenberg, G.J.; Cabeza, C.H.: Sudden hearing loss in divers and fliers. Laryngoscope *89:* 1373–1377 (1979).

Rask-Andersen, H.; Stahle, J.; Wilbrand, H.: Human cochlear aqueduct and its accessory canals. Ann. Otol. Rhinol. Lar. *86:* suppl. 42, pp. 1–16 (1977).

Ritter, F.N.; Lawrence, M.: A histological and experimental study of cochlear aqueduct patency in the adult human. Laryngoscope *75:* 1224–1233 (1965).

Rybak, L.P.: Perilymph fistula. Laryngoscope *90:* 2049–2050 (1980).

Simmons, F.B.: The double-membrane break syndrome in sudden hearing loss. Laryngoscope *89:* 59–66 (1979).

Sung, G.S.; Kamerer, D.B.; Sung, R.J.: Perilymphatic fistula and its interest to audiologists. J. Speech Hear. Disorders *41:* 540–546 (1976).

Terayama, Y.; Yamakawa, M.: Rupture of inner ear window, a case report. Otolaryngology, Tokyo *49:* 579–585 (1977).

Terayama, Y.; Yamakawa, M.; Nakamura, K.: Rupture of inner ear window. Pract. Otol., Kyoto *70:* 782–784 (1977).

Tingley, D.R.; MacDougall, J.A.: Round window tear in aviators. Aviat. Space envir. Med. *48:* 971–975 (1977).

Sekuta, J.; Wlodyka, J.: The round window in acute hearing loss. Audiology *21:* 55–60 (1982).

Weber-Liel: cited in Ahlén, G.: On the connection between cerebrospinal and intralabyrinthine pressure and pressure variations in the inner ear. Acta oto-lar. *35:* 251–257 (1947).

Weisskopf, A.; Murphy, J.T.; Merzenich, M.M.: Genesis of the round window rupture syndrome; some experimental observations. Laryngoscope *88:* 389–397 (1978).

Viral Labyrinthitis

Koide, J.; Kurata, T.; Hondo, R.: Experimental inner ear pathology with herpes simplex virus infection. 1. Intracerebral inoculation of herpes simplex virus in mice. J. Otolar. Jap. *85:* 288–292 (1982).

Kurata, T.; Koide, J.; Hondo, R., et al.: Herpes simplex virus (type 2) infection in the inner ear of the guinea pig. Annual Report of Idiopathic Sensorineural Hearing Loss, 1981, pp. 73–78 (Ministry of Welfare, Tokyo 1982).

Nomura, Y.: A model animal of viral type sudden deafness. Igaku no Ayumi *117:* 322–328 (1981).

Terayama, Y.; Tanaka, K.; Hirai, T.: An electron microscopic study of the cochlear nerve in viral labyrinthitis. Annual Report of Idiopathic Sensorineural Hearing Loss, 1979, pp. 17–19 (Ministry of Welfare, Tokyo 1980).

Otosclerosis (see chapt. 6)

Gisselsson, L.; Richter, O.: Ein Beitrag zur Frage des Hörvermögens bei Verschluss des runden Fensters. Arch. Ohrenheilk. *166:* 410–418 (1955).

Grant, H.: Round window occlusion in otosclerosis. J. Lar. Otol. *86:* 21–26 (1972).

Groen, J.J.; Hoogland, G.A.: Bone conduction and otosclerosis of the round window. Acta oto-lar. *49:* 206–212 (1958).

Guild, S.R.: Incidence, location and extent of otosclerotic lesions. Archs Otolar. *52:* 848–852 (1950).

Heermann, J., Jr.: Zur Chirurgie des runden Fensters bei Otosklerose. Z. Lar. Rhinol. Otol. *42:* 699–708 (1963).

Hoshino, T.; Kodama, A.; Toriyama, M.: Histological study of otosclerosis among the Japanese. Otolaryngology, Tokyo *48:* 547–552 (1976).

House, W.F.: Oval window and round window surgery in extensive otosclerosis. Laryngoscope *69:* 693–701 (1959).

House, W.F.; Glorig, A.: Criteria for otosclerosis surgery and further experiences with round window surgery. Laryngoscope *70:* 616–630 (1960).

Huygen, P.L.M.; Marres, E.H.M.A.; De Jong van de Brand, O.W.J.M.: Focus localization in two clinical types of otosclerosis. Acta oto-lar. *78:* 365–370 (1974).

Lindsay, J.R.; Hemenway, W.G.: Occlusion of the round window by otosclerosis. Laryngoscope *64:* 10–19 (1954).

Tonndorf, J.; Tabor, J.R.: Closure of the cochlear windows. Its effect upon air and bone conduction. Ann. Otol. Rhinol. Lar. *71:* 5–29 (1962).

Anomaly

Berézin, M.A.: Surdité congénitale de transmission par fermeture de la fenêtre ronde. Annls Oto-lar. *83:* 878–880 (1966).

Bernstein, L.: Congenital absence of the oval window. Archs Otolar. *83:* 533–537 (1966).

Caplinger, M.C.B.; Hora, M.J.F.: Middle ear choristoma with absent oval widow. Archs Otolar. *85:* 365–366 (1967).

Durcan, D.J.; Shea, J.J.; Sleeckx, J.P.: Bifurcation of the facial nerve. Archs Otolar. *86:* 619–631 (1967).

Everberg, G.: Congenital absence of the oval window. Acta oto-lar. *66:* 320–332 (1968).

Fernandez, A.O.; Ronis, M.L.: Congenital absence of the oval window: a review of the literature and report of a case. Laryngoscope *74:* 186–197 (1964).

Harada, T.; Black, F.O.; Sando, I.; Singleton, G.T.: Temporal bone histopathologic findings in congenital anomalies of the oval window. Otolar. Head Neck Surg. *88:* 275–287 (1980).

Harrison, W.H.; Shambaugh, G.E.; Derlacki, E.L.: Congenital absence of the round window: case report with surgical reconstruction by cochlear fenestration. Laryngoscope *74:* 967–978 (1964).

Hociotă, D.; Ataman, T.: A case of salivary gland choristoma of the middle ear. J. Lar. Otol. *89:* 1065–1068 (1975).

Hough, J.V.D.: Malformations and anatomical variations seen in the middle ear during the operation for mobilization of the stapes. Laryngoscope *68:* 1337–1379 (1958).

Jahrsdoerfer, R.A.: Congenital absence of the oval window. Trans. Am. Acad. Ophthal. Oto-lar. *84:* 904–914 (1977).

Krampitz, P.: Über einige seltenere Formen von Missbildungen des Gehörorgans. Z. Ohren-heilk. *65:* 44–54 (1912).

Livingstone, G.: The establishment of sound conduction in congenital deformities of the external ear. J. Lar. Otol. *73:* 231–241 (1959).

Livingstone, G.; Delahunty, J.E.: Malformation of the ear associated with congenital ophthalmic and other conditions. J. Lar. Otol. *82:* 495–504 (1968).

Nakamura, S.; Sando, I.: Congenital absence of oval window. J. Otolar. Jap. *68:* 1416–1422 (1965).

Nakano, Y.; Takashima, M.: Congenital absence of the two cochlear windows. Otolaryngology, Tokyo *41:* 3–9 (1969).

Ombredanne, M.: Chirurgie des 'aplasies mineures': ses resultats dans les grandes surdites congenitales par malformations ossiculaires. Annls Oto-lar. *81:* 201–222 (1964).

Ombredanne, M.: Absence congénitale de fenêtre ronde dans certaines aplasies mineures. Annls Oto-lar. *85:* 369–378 (1968).

Richards, S.H.: Congenital absence of the round window treated by cochlear fenestration. Clin. Otolaryngol. *6:* 265–269 (1981).

Sellars, S.L.; Beighton, P.H.: Deafness in osteodysplasty of Melnick and Needles. Archs Otolar. *104:* 225–227 (1978).

9. Via the Round Window Therapeutics for Ear Diseases
Ablation Therapy

Cawthorne, T.E.: The treatment of Ménière's disease. J. Lar. Otol. *58:* 363–371 (1943).

Kossoff, G.; Wadsworth, J.R.; Dudley, P.F.: The round window ultrasonic technique for treatment of Ménière's disease. Archs Otolar. *86:* 535–542 (1967).

Lempert, J.: Lempert decompression operation for hydrops of the endolymphatic labyrinth in Ménière's disease. Archs Otolar. *47:* 551–570 (1948).

Pappas, J.J.; Bailey, H.A.T., Jr.; Graham, S.S.: Round window ultrasonic irradiation: conservative surgery for Ménière's disease. Am. J. Otol. *1:* 88–93 (1980).

Schreiner, L.: Experimentelle Untersuchungen über die Bildungsstätten und den Stoffaustausch der Perilymphe. Acta oto-lar. *212:* suppl., pp. 1–56 (1966).

Schuknecht, H.F.: Ablation therapy in the management of Ménière's disease. Acta oto-lar. *132:* suppl., pp. 1–42 (1957).

Schuknecht, H.; Hammerschlag, P.: Transcanal labyrinthectomy; in Silverstein, Norell, Neurological surgery of the ear, p. 172 (Aesculapius, Birmingham 1977).

Osmotic Induction Therapy

Arslan, M.: Modification of the osmotic pressure of perilymph and endolymph. Hypothesis on the pathogenesis of Ménière's disease. Acta oto-lar. *67:* 360–377 (1969).

Arslan, M.: Choice of surgical procedure in Ménière's disease. Proposal for a new osmotic 'induction' method. J. Lar. Otol. *84:* 131–147 (1970).

Arslan, M.: Treatment of Ménière's disease by application of sodium chloride crystals on the round window. Laryngoscope *82:* 1736–1750 (1972).

Asakuma, S.; Nakajima, T.; Matsumoto, I., et al.: Modification of endocochlear DC potential and histological changes of inner ear by NaCl crystals administered on round window membrane. Otol. Fukuoka *19:* 759–764 (1973).

Egami, T.; Nakajima, S.; Miyazaki, M., et al.: Positional nystagmus induced by infusion of saturated NaCl solution into the tympanic cavity. Pract. Otol., Kyoto *75:* suppl. 1, pp. 150–155 (1982).

Fowler, E.P., Jr.; Forbes, T.W.: End-organ deafness in dogs due to the application of certain chemicals to the round window membrane. Ann. Otol. Rhinol. Lar. *45:* 859–864 (1936).

Futaki, T.; Morimoto, M.; Yoza, T.: Effect of furosemide on nystagmus produced by applying NaCl crystals on the rabbit round window. Annual Report of Idiopathic Sensorineural Hearing Loss, 1979, pp. 151–156 (Ministry of Welfare, Tokyo 1980).

Hirashima, N.: Effect of prednisolone upon cochlear microphonics modified by NaCl crystals application to the round window membrane. Otol. Fukuoka *22:* 45–50 (1976).

Molinari, G.A.: Alterations of inner ear mechanisms resulting from application of sodium chloride to the round window membrane. Ann. Otol. Rhinol. Lar. *81:* 315–322 (1972).

Cochlear Endolymphatic Shunt (Cochleosacculotomy)

Cody, D.T.R.: The tack operation for endolymphatic hydrops. Laryngoscope *79:* 1737–1744 (1969).

Cody, D.T.R.; Simonton, K.M.; Hallberg, O.E.: Automatic repetitive decompression of the saccule in endolymphatic hydrops (tack operation). Preliminary report. Laryngoscope *77:* 1480–1501 (1967).

Fick, I.A. van N.: Decompression of the labyrinth. A new surgical procedure for Ménière's disease. Archs Otolar. *79:* 447–458 (1964).

Fick, I.A. van N.: Ménière's disease: aetiology and a new surgical approach: sacculotomy. J. Lar. Otol. *80:* 288–306 (1966).

Nomura, Y.: Surgery of the round window. Otolaryngology, Tokyo *54:* 969–972 (1982).

Nomura, Y.; Futaki, T.; Fukaya, T.: Cochleosacculotomy. Otolaryngology, Tokyo *55:* 245–259 (1983).

Pulec, J.L.: The otic-perotic shunt. Otol. Clins N. Am. *1:* 643–648 (1968).

Pulec, J.L.; The surgical treatment of vertigo. Laryngoscope *79:* 1783–1822 (1969).

Schuknecht, H.F.: Rationale of surgical procedures for Ménière's disease; in Vosteen, Schuknecht, Pfaltz, Wersäll, Kimura, Morgenstern, Juhn, Ménière's disease, pp. 236–242 (Thieme, Stuttgart 1981).

Schuknecht, H.F.: Cochleosacculotomy for Ménière's disease: theory, technique and results. Laryngoscope *92:* 853–858 (1982).

Singular Neurectomy

Epley, J.M.: Singular neurectomy: hypotympanotomy approach. Otolar. Head Neck Surg. *88:* 304–309 (1980).

Gacek, R.R.: Transection of the posterior ampullary nerve for the relief of benign paroxysmal positional vertigo. Ann. Otol. Rhinol. Lar. *83:* 596–605 (1974).

Gacek, R.R.: Further observations on posterior ampullary nerve transection for positional vertigo. Ann. Otol. Rhinol. Lar. *87:* 300–305 (1978).
Okano, Y.; Sando, I.; Myers, E.N.: Branch of the singular nerve (posterior ampullary nerve)
    in the otic capsule. Ann. Otol. Rhinol. Lar. *89:* 13–19 (1980).
Schuknecht, H.F.: Cupulolithiasis. Archs Otolar. *90:* 765–778 (1969).

Subject Index